Effective Communication in Veterinary Medicine

Editors

CHRISTOPHER A. ADIN
KELLY D. FARNSWORTH

VETERINARY CLINICS OF NORTH AMERICA: SMALL ANIMAL PRACTICE

www.vetsmall.theclinics.com

September 2021 • Volume 51 • Number 5

ELSEVIER

1600 John F. Kennedy Boulevard ● Suite 1800 ● Philadelphia, Pennsylvania, 19103-2899
http://www.vetsmall.theclinics.com

VETERINARY CLINICS OF NORTH AMERICA: SMALL ANIMAL PRACTICE Volume 51, Number 5
September 2021 ISSN 0195-5616, ISBN-13: 978-0-323-89746-4

Editor: Stacy Eastman
Developmental Editor: Axell Ivan Jade Purificacion

Veterinary Clinics of North America: Small Animal Practice (ISSN 0195-5616) is published bimonthly by Elsevier Inc., 360
Park Avenue South, New York, NY 10010-1710. Months of issue are January, March, May, July, September, and
November. Business and Editorial Offices: 1600 John F. Kennedy Blvd., Ste. 1800, Philadelphia, PA 19103-2899.
Customer Service Office: 3251 Riverport Lane, Maryland Heights, MO 63043. Periodicals postage paid at New York,
NY and additional mailing offices. Subscription prices are $358.00 per year (domestic individuals), $933.00 per year
(domestic institutions), $100.00 per year (domestic students/residents), $451.00 per year (Canadian individuals),
$998.00 per year (Canadian institutions), $488.00 per year (international individuals), $998.00 per year (international
institutions), $100.00 per year (Canadian students/residents), and $220.00 per year (international students/residents).
To receive student/resident rate, orders must be accompanied by name of affiliated institution, date of term, and the *sig-
nature* of program/residency coordinator on institution letterhead. Orders will be billed at individual rate until proof of status
is received. Foreign air speed delivery is included in all *Clinics* subscription prices. All prices are subject to change without
notice. **POSTMASTER:** Send address changes to *Veterinary Clinics of North America: Small Animal Practice*, Elsevier
Health Sciences Division, Subscription Customer Service, 3251 Riverport Lane, Maryland Heights, MO 63043. Customer
Service (orders, claims, online, change of address): Elsevier Periodicals Customer Service, Elsevier Health Sciences Di-
vision Subscription **Customer Service 3251 Riverport Lane Maryland Heights, MO 63043. Tel: 1-800-654-2452
(U.S. and Canada); 314-447-8871 (outside U.S. and Canada). Fax: 314-447-8029. E-mail: journalscustomerser-
vice-usa@elsevier.com (for print support); journalsonlinesupport-usa@elsevier.com (for online support).**
Reprints. For copies of 100 or more of articles in this publication, please contact the Commercial Reprints Department,
Elsevier Inc., 360 Park Avenue South, New York, NY 10010-1710. Tel.: 212-633-3874; Fax: 212-633-3820; E-mail:
reprints@elsevier.com.

Veterinary Clinics of North America: Small Animal Practice is also published in Japanese by Inter Zoo Publishing
Co., Ltd., Aoyama Crystal-Bldg 5F, 3-5-12 Kitaaoyama, Minato-ku, Tokyo 107-0061, Japan.

Veterinary Clinics of North America: Small Animal Practice is covered in *Current Contents/Agriculture, Biology and Environmental Sciences, Science Citation Index, ASCA, MEDLINE/PubMed (Index Medicus), Excerpta Medica, and BIOSIS.*

Contributors

EDITORS

CHRISTOPHER A. ADIN, DVM
Diplomate, American College of Veterinary Surgeons; Professor and Chair, Department of Small Animal Clinical Sciences, College of Veterinary Medicine, University of Florida, Gainesville, Florida, USA

KELLY D. FARNSWORTH, DVM, MS
Diplomate, American College of Veterinary Surgeons; Clinical Associate Professor in Equine Surgery, Department of Clinical Sciences, College of Veterinary Medicine, Washington State University, Pullman, Washington, USA

AUTHORS

CHRISTOPHER A. ADIN, DVM
Diplomate, American College of Veterinary Surgeons; Professor and Chair, Department of Small Animal Clinical Sciences, College of Veterinary Medicine, University of Florida, Gainesville, Florida, USA

ELIZABETH M. CHARLES, DVM, MA
Executive Director, Veterinary Leadership Institute, Adjunct Faculty, Lincoln Memorial University, CEO, Radiology, Rules, Temecula, California, USA

BETH DAVIDOW, DVM
Diplomate, American College Veterinary Emergency and Critical Care; Clinical Assistant Professor, Veterinary Clinical Sciences, Washington State University, Pullman, Washington, USA

YVONNE ELCE, DVM
Diplomate, American College of Veterinary Surgeons; Associate Professor, Atlantic Veterinary College, University of PEI, Charlottetown, Prince Edward Island, Canada

KELLY D. FARNSWORTH, DVM, MS
Diplomate, American College of Veterinary Surgeons; Clinical Associate Professor in Equine Surgery, Department of Clinical Sciences, College of Veterinary Medicine, Washington State University, Pullman, Washington, USA

CALLIE FOGLE, DVM
Diplomate, American College of Veterinary Surgeons; Clinical Professor, Equine Surgery, Department of Clinical Sciences, North Carolina State University, Raleigh, North Carolina, USA

KELLY HARRISON, DVM, MS
University of Florida College of Veterinary Medicine, Gainesville, Florida, USA

JOANNE INTILE, DVM, MS
Diplomate, American College of Veterinary Internal Medicine; Associate Clinical
Professor, Medical Oncology, Department of Clinical Sciences, North Carolina State
University, Raleigh, North Carolina, USA

MAGGIE G. MORTALI, MPH
Senior Program Director, American Foundation for Suicide Prevention, New York, New
York, USA

CHRISTINE MOUTIER, MD
Chief Medical Officer, American Foundation for Suicide Prevention, New York, New York,
USA

ZENITHSON Y. NG, DVM, MS
Diplomate, American Board of Veterinary Practitioners (Canine and Feline); Clinical
Associate Professor, Department of Small Animal Clinical Sciences, The University of
Tennessee, Knoxville, Tennessee, USA

ADESOLA ODUNAYO, DVM, MS
Diplomate, American College of Veterinary Emergency and Critical Care; Clinical
Associate Professor, Department of Small Animal Clinical Sciences, The University of
Tennessee, Knoxville, Tennessee, USA

MARY KATHERINE SHEATS, DVM, PhD
Diplomate, American College of Veterinary Internal Medicine; Assistant Professor, Equine
Primary Care, Department of Clinical Sciences, North Carolina State University, Raleigh,
North Carolina, USA

Contents

A Strategy for Effective Generational Communication in Veterinary Medicine   985

Elizabeth M. Charles and Kelly D. Farnsworth

> In today's veterinary practices, 5 generations (traditionalists, baby boomers, Generation X, millennials, and Generation Z), each with a unique way of looking at the world, are trying to work together effectively. Common strategies for managing this multigenerational workplace include villainizing "other" generations or merely tolerating their presence. Conflict, disagreements, and misunderstanding often get in the way of practicing quality medicine. Thus, veterinary health professionals must develop strategies that allow for effective communication, not only within the practice but also with clients, vendors, and other stakeholders, a strategy that builds bridges among the generations through engagement, regardless of generation.

Challenges in Intercultural Communication   999

Kelly D. Farnsworth

> With the increasing diversity of our clients or potential clients it is important for us as veterinary professionals to recognize the opportunities this affords us to serve a larger demographic. However, along with this opportunity comes the challenges of serving clients for whom English may be a second language as well as clients who may have very different understanding of health care options for their animal. By seeking to become more culturally aware, we can have significant impact on the care of our patients. This article focuses on both awareness and skills to aid this process.

Valuing Diversity in the Team   1009

Adesola Odunayo and Zenithson Y. Ng

> One of the most impactful ways to create a dynamic team is to foster diversity and inclusivity within the workplace. Workplaces have become more heterogenous as advances in human, women, and civil rights group have spurred greater labor force participation by members of historically underrepresented groups. Studies have shown that leveraging diversity has important implications for the promotion of positive organization change through facilitation of individual and organization performance. Diverse clientele may be more comfortable and feel more welcome working with people in a diverse workplace.

VETERINARY CLINICS OF NORTH AMERICA: SMALL ANIMAL PRACTICE

FORTHCOMING ISSUES

November 2021
Diagnostic Imaging: Point-of-Care Ultrasound
Gregory R. Lisciandro and Jennifer M. Gambino, *Editors*

January 2022
Veterinary Dentistry and Oral Surgery
Alexander M. Reiter, *Editor*

March 2022
Soft Tissue Surgery
Nicole J. Buote, *Editor*

RECENT ISSUES

July 2021
Working Dogs: An Update for Veterinarians
Maureen A. McMichael, Melissa Singletary, *Editors*

May 2021
Small Animal Nutrition
Dottie Laflamme, *Editor*

March 2021
Forelimb Lameness
Kevin Benjamino and Kenneth A. Bruecker, *Editors*

SERIES OF RELATED INTEREST

Veterinary Clinics of North America: Exotic Animal Practice
https://www.vetexotic.theclinics.com/

THE CLINICS ARE NOW AVAILABLE ONLINE!
Access your subscription at:
www.theclinics.com

Erratum

In the article, "Nutritional Management for Dogs and Cats with Chronic Kidney Disease," by Valerie J. Parker, published in the May 2021 issue (Volume 51, number 3, pages 685-710), in Table 3 on page 12, for the "2020 AAFCO Feline adult maintenance maximum requirement" under the "Vitamin D (IU)", the correct number should be 752 instead of 75.2.

Vet Clin Small Anim 51 (2021) ix
https://doi.org/10.1016/j.cvsm.2021.07.014

Preface

Communications Training: The Next Level

To effectively communicate, we must realize that we are all different in the way we perceive the world and use this understanding as a guide to our communication with others.

—*Tony Robbins*

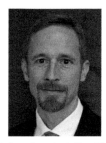 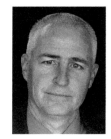

Christopher A. Adin, DVM   Kelly D. Farnsworth, DVM, MS

Editors

Veterinary medicine has changed significantly since the *Veterinary Clinics of North America: Small Animal Practice* dedicated its first issue to the topic of communication in 2007. At that time, early adopters had recognized the importance of communication skills in veterinary practice, and their efforts contributed to the incorporation of communications training into the accreditation standards of the American Veterinary Medical Association (AVMA) for the veterinary curriculum. Now, veterinary students in AVMA accredited schools around the world are graduating with training in the use of core skills like reflective listening, open-ended questions, expression of empathy, and the use of nonverbal communication. The majority of veterinarians will also have had the opportunity to obtain training in specific topics, such as end-of-life decisions, financial discussions, conflict negotiation, and team building. With this background in mind, the current issue moves beyond the core techniques that have permeated the veterinary profession and presents timely guidance on how small animal practitioners can apply their growing communication skills to the important challenges that they face today. Readers will find pertinent information on generational communication, intercultural communication, valuing diversity, compassion fatigue, suicide warning signs and interventions, difficult performance evaluations, change management, clinical ethics, mentorship, and patient quality and safety.

Electric communication will never be a substitute for the face of someone who with their soul encourages another person to be brave and true.

—*Charles Dickens*

Vet Clin Small Anim 51 (2021) xi–xii
https://doi.org/10.1016/j.cvsm.2021.06.001
0195-5616/21/© 2021 Published by Elsevier Inc.

Another important change that had occurred since the last issue of *Veterinary Clinics of North America: Small Animal Practice* was dedicated to communication is the widespread use of social media and electronic forms of communication. In the quotation above, Charles Dickens (1812-1870) showed incredible precognition of the problems that society would face when electronic communication superseded direct communication with another human being. While mass communication and social media have the potential to bring people together and to influence change, small animal practitioners will continue to need and use direct communication with clients, staff, and coworkers from different backgrounds. Our commitment to this idea is reflected not only in the topics of the articles in this issue but also in the diverse backgrounds of the authors that have shared their experiences and ideas. We look forward to seeing how our profession can unite in using excellent communication to meet the challenges of the next decade.

Christopher A. Adin, DVM
Department of Small Animal Clinical Sciences
College of Veterinary Medicine
University of Florida
PO Box 100162
Gainesville, FL 32610-0162, USA

Kelly D. Farnsworth, DVM, MS
Department of Clinical Sciences
College of Veterinary Medicine
Washington State University
100 Grimes Way
Pullman, WA 99163, USA

E-mail addresses:
adinc@ufl.edu (C.A. Adin)
farns005@wsu.edu (K.D. Farnsworth)

A Strategy for Effective Generational Communication in Veterinary Medicine

Elizabeth M. Charles, DVM, MA[a],*, Kelly Farnsworth, DVM, MS[b,1]

KEYWORDS

- Generation • Effective communication • Veterinary medicine • Engagement
- Self-awareness • Self-management • Social awareness • Relationship management

KEY POINTS

- Effective generational communication, decreased generational bias, learning how to speak other generation's language, building cross-generational relationships.
- Understanding generational differences leads to more effective communication and teamwork.
- The emotional intelligence framework of self-awareness, self-management, social awareness and relationship management is critical to effective generational communication.
- Though understanding generational biases is important, it is not the only factor necessary for successful teamwork within veterinary practice.

"[Young people] have exalted notions, because they have not yet been humbled by life or learnt its necessary limitations; moreover, their hopeful disposition makes them think themselves equal to great things—and that means having exalted notions."[1]

—*Aristotle*

INTRODUCTION

It is tempting to think the current generation gap is unique to present-day experience. Young people today are entitled and so sure of themselves, and it is nearly impossible to work with them. Old people are stuck in their ways and unwilling to change, and it is nearly impossible to work with them. Somehow it seems this generation is facing something that no other generations in history have faced. Unfortunately, as Aristotle's thoughts so perfectly illustrate, as long as there have been people, older people have

---

[a] Veterinary Leadership Institute, Lincoln Memorial University, RadiologyRules, PO Box 1476, Temecula, CA 92591, USA; [b] Department of Veterinary Clinical Sciences, Washington State University, Pullman, WA, USA
[1] Present address: 8002 Dry Creek Road, Garfield, WA 99130.
* Corresponding author.
E-mail address: betsycharles@mac.com

Vet Clin Small Anim 51 (2021) 985–997
https://doi.org/10.1016/j.cvsm.2021.05.001
0195-5616/21/© 2021 Elsevier Inc. All rights reserved.

vetsmall.theclinics.com

taken issue with the "confidence" young people bring to the table despite their lack of experience or understanding of how the world works. Young people are still full of naïve enthusiasm associated with changing the world for the better without a nod to the experience of their elders. Aristotle gives some evidence that the communication struggles of those who came before are no different than the communication struggles of today. Present-day researchers continue to support that same assertion, as Wen and colleagues[2] found tension in the workplace often is a concern when multiple generations are trying to work together.

The generation gap has always existed. Ultimately, the size of the gap is determined by myriad factors, including internal factors like personality, stage in life, responses to stress, what is happening in society, and how individuals process information, conflict management styles, and preferred communication approaches.[3,4] External factors like socioeconomic status, the way one is raised, the part of the country one grows up in, and how the collective cohort responds to societal circumstances also play a role in shaping who we are.[5] If this is the case, how can the gap be closed so that veterinary teams can work together effectively? Before moving into a discussion about the strategy for effective generational communication, an introduction to how each generation is defined, a brief overview of some of the filters used in generational research, and historical context for how the strategy was developed are in order.

Currently, 3 generations, the baby boomers, Generation X, and the millennials, each with their own unique way of looking at the world, are trying to work together and collaborate to provide exceptional veterinary service to clients. Add to that mix a handful of remaining traditionalists and the first wave of Generation Z starting to enter the workforce, and it is understandable why there is an epic clash of generations in the workforce.[6] It is not unusual for conflict, disagreements, and misunderstanding to get in the way of practicing quality medicine. Thus, it is important for veterinary professionals to develop a strategy and skill set that allows for effective communication, not only within the practice but also with clients, vendors, and other valuable stakeholders—a strategy that builds bridges among the generations and engages all members of the team, regardless of their generation.[7]

As discussed previously, the generation into which we were born is only part of the story that makes us, us. Many factors play a role in shaping how each person moves through the world. Exceptions to the rule, however, always exist. The information presented about each generation is based on the research and the trends identified within that research (**Fig. 1**), but outliers abound. Not everyone fits neatly into their generational box. Essentially, the words of Alexandre Dumas must be heeded: All generalizations are dangerous, even this one.

Generation	Born	Age in 2020	Tech
Traditionalists	1928–1945	75–92	Typewriter
Baby boomers	1946–1964	56–74	Mainframe
Generation X	1965–1980	40–55	PC
Millennials	1981–1996	24–39	Internet
Generation Z	1997–2012	8–23	Wearable tech

Fig. 1. A summary of the current generations working together in veterinary medicine.

GENERATIONAL OVERVIEW

The traditionalists were born prior to 1946 and were faced with myriad adversities during their formative years, including firsthand experience with the Great Depression and its aftermath as well as World War II. They grew up in an environment where "right" and "wrong" were defined clearly by their parents and a strong work ethic was what led to prosperity. A woman's place was in the home, raising the children, while it was the man's responsibility to provide for the family financially, and children were best seen and not heard.[4,8,9] From a technology standpoint, traditionalists came of age with the typewriter and radio.[10]

The baby boomers were born from 1946 to 1964 and came of age during the thriving new economy that followed World War II, which led this generation to be very secure and optimistic. They experienced the shift from the golden age of radio to television as well as a move from the country into suburbia. As a result, they learned about values not only from their families but also from television and their neighbors. With security came an outward focus that caused them to question the status quo leading to the civil rights and women's movements as well as antiwar sentiment specifically targeted at the Vietnam War. Due to their numbers, the workplace was very competitive.[4,8,9] From a technology standpoint, baby boomers came of age with the mainframe computer.[10]

Generation X was born from 1965 to 1980 and, unlike their baby boomer parents, were born into a world of uncertainty and turmoil as civil rights and women's liberation, political scandal, inflation, and massive corporate layoffs led to an environment of distrust and fear. Because both Dad and Mom were at work, the resulting latchkey kids came home to an empty house after school and learned to be independent and resourceful. After watching their parents get laid off and then divorced, they are skeptical of the way things have always been done and are more interested in working to live, rather than living to work, the first generation to emphasize work-life balance.[4,8,9] From a technology standpoint, Generation X came of age with personal computers.[10]

The millennials were born from 1981 to 1999 and came into the world at a time of unprecedented growth and prosperity and are struggling to understand how to function in a world that is now facing economic crisis. Raised by helicopter parents who hovered over their every move, this generation is very confident and has been told by their parents and teachers they can be whatever they want to be.[11] They may have vague memories of life without the Internet, but they are fluent in its language. They have experienced adversity through the lens of the media thanks to 24-hour news coverage by CNN. They are an incredibly diverse generation and they do not understand the need for diversity training.[4,8,9,12] From a technology standpoint, millennials came of age with smartphones.[10]

Generation Z members started to hit the ground in 1997. The closing end of this generation has yet to be solidified, but many report the end as 2012. They are truly digital natives and do not know life without the Internet. They have no clue that phones ever were actually attached to the wall. Author Tim Elmore[13] describes this generation as overwhelmed, overconnected, overprotected, and overserved, all things that have led to a lack of development of healthy coping strategies, interpersonal skills, and relationship skills as well as increased levels of anxiety and depression. On the flip side, they also are energetic, passionate about changing the world, confident, and capable.[13,14] They are well on their way to becoming the largest generation.[15] They are like the millennials, with smartphones and wearable technology like smart watches shaping how they interact with the world.[12]

GENERATIONAL RESEARCH OVERVIEW

It is beyond the scope of this article to review all the pros and cons associated with putting people into categories based on when they were born and the research challenges posed by doing so. People are complex and the forces that shape attitudes, behaviors, work ethic, and communication style are many and multifactorial. It is helpful, however, to have a basic understanding of the factors that must be considered when doing generational research. According to the Pew Research Center, "An individual's age is one of the most common predictors of differences in attitudes and behaviors."[3] Several different strategies are used to understand generational tendencies and trends associated with a generation's attitudes and behaviors. Inherent in these strategies is the difficulty with isolating specific factors and identifying their individual influence on generational differences, so acknowledging the interplay between factors is critical. In general, life cycle or age effect, period effect, and cohort effect all can play a role in how a generation of people develop.[3]

Life cycle or age effect takes into consideration the fact that the things that matter to people when they are in their 20s are not necessarily the things that matter to them when they are in their 40s or 70s. We are, in many ways, a product of the stage of life we are in, and priorities, in general, reflect what matters during different life stages. Period effect considers that larger societal circumstances play a role in determining how we show up in the world, especially if those circumstances take place during the formative years. At the time of publication of this issue of *Veterinary Clinics of North America*, we will be entering the second year of a global pandemic associated with COVID-19 that changed life as we know it. This is a perfect example of the period effect on a generation and the ramifications for Generation Z on their outlook, attitudes, and behaviors will be interesting to study. Other examples include the Vietnam War for baby boomers, the space shuttle Challenger explosion for Generation X, and 9/11 for millennials. The cohort effect is when 1 generation experiences something as a group that the other generations have not experienced.[3]

COMMUNICATION STRATEGY DEVELOPMENT

Dr Charles, a poster child for Generation X, began exploring the topic of generational communication in veterinary medicine because she was struggling to communicate effectively with her boss and mentor, himself a poster child for the baby boomers. Her personal communication challenges led to advanced training in organizational leadership and then a shift in jobs to a position teaching veterinary students, where she was given daily opportunities to manage the generation gap. Over the course of 7 years as a faculty member managing communication between millennial students and Generation X/boomer faculty members, she developed this strategy. It is the result of years of reading in diverse disciplines like emotional intelligence, hostage negotiations, communication (specifically, challenging conversations), conflict resolution, influence, and leadership and combining specific skills sets into a cohesive approach to closing the generational communication gap. The strategy foundation? Emotional intelligence.

In their 1990 article, Peter Salovey and John Mayer[16] coined the term, *emotional intelligence*, and began an organized and scientific approach to better understand how emotions contribute to intelligence and success. Their work, although groundbreaking and critically important, was difficult to apply to the real world in a meaningful manner. Enter Daniel Goleman.[17] He streamlined and packaged the concepts for the lay audience, while popularizing the term, *EQ*, to describe this "other" intelligence that is so critical to success. In his 1998 article, "What Makes a Leader?" he outlined the 5 components of emotional intelligence: self-awareness, self-regulation, motivation, empathy, and social skill.[17] The generational communication strategy outlined in this paper is built on Salovey, Mayer, and Goleman's work but uses the simple emotional intelligence framework (self-awareness, self-management, social awareness, and relationship management) outlined by Travis Bradberry and Jean Greaves in their book, *Emotional Intelligence 2.0*.[18] Self-awareness, or the ability to understand one's own weaknesses and strengths as well as the lenses through which one looks when interacting with others, is an essential starting place for effective communication and interaction. Self-management is the ability to suspend judgment and control responses to situations to have a fair and healthy outcome. Social awareness deals with the ability to relate to others such that one considers the other person's situation, background, and feelings before an interaction occurs.[16–18] Finally, relationship management involves putting it all together in such a way that the desired outcomes are achieved, or, as Goleman puts it, "friendliness with a purpose."[17] Applying these concepts to the generation gap provides an effective strategy for multi-generational communication and interaction (**Fig. 2**).

The remainder of this article describes each step of the strategy through an example story to set the stage, identification of some of the skills sets necessary to successfully navigate the example, and a closing assignment to allow the reader to practice 1 or more of the skills used in the story. Although this article focuses on using this strategy as it applies to generational communication, the strategy also applies to any communication that involves diversity of opinion or experience.

Step 1: Recognize Your Own Generational Bias (Self-Awareness)

Although conflicting research exists concerning the significance of the generation gap among the generations,[9] understanding what, in general, has shaped one's own generation (self-awareness) as well as what has shaped the other generations (social awareness, discussed later) is a helpful starting point for making sure interactions among members of each generation are positive and not wrought with assumptions and tension.[19] This step often is the most difficult one because it forces self-reflection, something

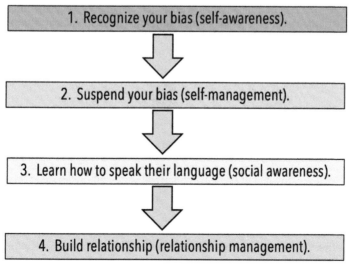

Fig. 2. Overview of the generational communication strategy.

most high performing individuals in demanding careers like veterinary medicine do not put into the schedule. It also requires an open-minded approach to other people's generational lenses. Often, each generation makes the assumption that the way they did things was not only the right way but also the best way. Thus, the first step requires recognizing that we have a generational bias. Awareness of this bias leads to better understanding that the way one generation looks at the world is not necessarily right or wrong, it is just different.

Consider this interaction between Dr Smith, the supervisor of an equine imaging center, and a second-year student, Sarah, visiting Dr Smith's practice for a 2-week externship.

Dr Smith spent approximately 10 minutes explaining how each morning would start during the externship. Sarah would arrive by 8:00 AM and perform physical examinations on each of the horses in the clinic (capacity for the clinic = 10 horses) and then report those findings in the patients' medical records. Dr Smith was barely finished with her explanation when Sarah let out a big sigh, rolled her eyes, and said, "I don't understand why I have to do physical exams on basically healthy horses. I mean they are all here for some sort of lameness issue. It's not like they are sick." Dr Smith felt her face flush and her heart start pounding. Without skipping a beat, she shot back as she pointed to the barn a short distance from where she and the student were standing, "When I was in vet school, we didn't talk to our professors like that. If you want to pass this rotation, you get your butt up there to the barn and do the physical exams." Sarah crossed her arms, spun around, and stomped her way up to the barn.

Time out!! Before we go any further, stop and think about the biases Dr Smith is bringing to the table about her millennial student as well as the biases the student has toward her Generation X supervisor (**Fig. 3**).

Both people in the conversation are making assumptions about the other, likely based on the words used and nonverbal behaviors as well as opinions about why older people do the things they do and why younger people do the things they do. Both Dr Smith and Sarah need to recognize they are wearing their own generational glasses and that fact has led to a negative interaction.

What skills sets are required to recognize generational biases? Self-awareness is a must and, in this scenario, it can be broken down into 4 parts: (1) pay attention to your physiology, (2) name the emotion you are feeling, (3) ask why—Why are you feeling the emotion you are feeling? and (4) take a moment for reflection (usually after the fact). A physiologic response usually is one of the first clues that something is not going well in a conversation and often can be linked to the fight/flight/freeze stress response.[20] Sarah's sigh coupled with an eye roll signals possible frustration/annoyance at being asked to do physical examinations on what she thought were essentially healthy

Dr. Smith's Biases	Sarah's Biases
Sarah is lazy and entitled.	Dr. Smith is really bossy.
Sarah does not have a good work ethic.	Dr. Smith is lazy as she wants the students
Sarah is disrespectful of her elders.	to do her dirty work.
Sarah is unwilling to learn.	Dr. Smith likes to power trip.
Sarah does not understand her place on	Dr. Smith is not a good teacher.
the team as an extern.	Dr. Smith has an anger management
Sarah thinks she knows everything.	problem.

Fig. 3. In each box, 1 for Dr Smith and 1 for Sarah, possible biases are listed for each person. They both come to the interaction with a specific lens through which they look when it comes to stereotypes or biases about other generations. These are just a few possibilities for each person.

horses.[11] She did not recognize her biases and, therefore, could not suspend them (discussed later), so she responded in a less than professional manner by sighing and rolling her eyes. Dr Smith also failed to acknowledge the emotions her biases caused and suspend them so she, too, responded in an inappropriate way by barking orders at Sarah.

To better understand one's own generational bias, consider the following questions. Why do I have a problem with the older/younger generations? What is it that bothers me about my associate's desire to have work-life balance? Can I explain the benefit of "paying your dues?" What threats do traditionalist/baby boomer/Generation X/millennial values represent? What role do I play in causing the tension between us? How will I need to change in order to take advantage of the generation opportunity instead of increasing the generation gap? Why do I get so frustrated when my boss doesn't acknowledge my new ideas?

Self-awareness is a skill that can be practiced and will help not only with generational communication but also with many other things because it is the foundation of emotional intelligence. By paying attention to your physiology, learning how to name the emotions you are feeling, understanding the why underneath those emotions and taking time to reflect on what you are learning about yourself, you will become more proficient in making sure your interactions are positive and intentional.[18]

Assignment: read each of the following scenarios (**Fig. 4**). Pay attention to what happens in your physiology as you read the scenario and consider the question at the end of the scenario. Name the emotions that result from reading the scenario. Ask yourself why you feel the way you do (consider what is underneath the emotions). Spend a couple minutes reflecting on the experience using some of the previous questions.

Step 2: Suspend Your Generational Bias (Self-Management)

Much of the conflict that happens among generations is not grounded in fact but actually is based on assumption or, as discussed previously, generational biases. The

Scenario #1	You are the attending clinician at a large referral practice and are leading a discussion during rounds about a case. You look up and see one of your interns looking down at her phone, typing something and seemingly not engaged in the conversation. As the attending clinician, how do you handle this situation?
Scenario #2	You just get to class and sit down. The professor walks into the room and stands at the podium. The first thing he says is, "Please close your computers. I want you to actually listen to what I am teaching instead of surfing the web or updating your status." How does this make you feel?
Scenario #3	You are the professor of the large animal medicine rotation. It is your responsibility to set up the student emergency on-call schedule for the upcoming 4-week rotation. It is not uncommon for you to overhear students making comments like, "If this is how much I have to be on call, I'm not sure this is going to work for me," or "How am I supposed to have a life if I am on-call so much?" How do you, as the professor, turn this situation into a win-win for all involved?
Scenario #4	You were hired as an associate veterinary right out of veterinary school into a local equine practice that has been in busines for over 50 years. You have recently become the supervisor of the practice's social media endeavors, a job you enjoy and believe adds value to the practice. In order to do your job efficiently, high speed internet access is a must, something you have at home, but do not have at the practice due to the practice's location on the outskirts of the rural community it serves. Tension is increasing between you and your boss because you would like to take care of your social media responsibilities at home and then come to the clinic while your boss would like you in the office by 7:30am so you can be available should something "come up." How do you handle this situation?

Fig. 4. Use these scenarios to practice the skill of self-awareness.

difficulty with assumption as it pertains to generational issues goes back to one generation or another being right versus wrong, instead of just different. Each generation assumes its approach to life is the correct approach and then, if not able to suspend that bias, further assumes that anything the other generations do, say, and so forth, must be wrong.[21] Right versus wrong often can be emotionally charged and lead to negative interactions because from acting reflexively (limbic system/amygdala hijack) instead of rationally and with intention (frontal cortex).[20]

Going back to Dr Smith and Sarah, both parties did not practice the skill of self-management in their interaction. Instead of taking time to get her frontal cortex online so she could response thoughtfully, Sarah sighed and rolled her eyes, both paraverbal actions that often communicate disrespect. Dr Smith also neglected to take a moment to engage her rational mind and instead blurted out a totally inappropriate order to her student. Which skill set is required to avoid the situation that Dr Smith and her student found themselves in? The ability to self-manage so you can direct your behavior in a constructive manner. Viktor Frankl described self-management beautifully when he said, "Between stimulus and response there is a space. In that space is our opportunity to choose how we respond." Self-management is the ability to get into that space before responding (**Fig. 5**). But how is that done?

Several strategies that can be used to get into the space include, but are not limited to, tactical breathing, getting comfortable being uncomfortable, and staying curious.[22] Tactical breathing is a simple breathing technique that gives you time and gives the brain oxygen so the frontal cortex can be engaged. It involves breathing in over a count of 4, holding the breath for a count of 4, exhaling to a count of 4, and holding the breath for a count of 4. This cycle is repeated as many times as is necessary to manage the body's attempts to act without thinking.[23] While breathing, feelings can be acknowledged and recognized, which often are uncomfortable. When the frontal cortex is engaged successfully, the temptation to avoid the uncomfortable is reduced, so staying out of the comfort zone can be practiced, a place where growth and learning take place.[24]

Finally, when squarely in the space with the rational mind engaged, you can practice the skill of staying curious, because when we are curious, we can more readily learn about different perspectives. Older generations have much to learn from younger generations and vice versa. Cultivating curiosity opens the door for cross-generational learning. Chris Meyer at Atomic Object, a software design company, developed a great list of criteria for help stay curious: enter interactions with a clear and open mind, ask questions, become familiar with encountering the unfamiliar, diversify interests, and allow being amazed by everyday things.[25]

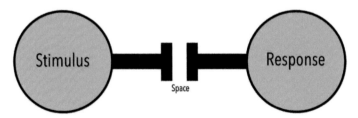

Fig. 5. This figure is a pictorial representation of Viktor Frankl's quotation that is referenced in the text. It is intended to help the reader better understand how to choose self-management by recognizing the space that allows practicing the skill of overriding the fight, flight, freeze response.

Although Dr Smith missed her first opportunity to get into the space while the interaction was happening with her student, she had time to re-evaluate her response after work and decided to have a conversation with Sarah the following morning. She began by asking questions and staying curious: "We had an interaction yesterday that did not go so well. You seemed frustrated with having to do physical exams on the horses in the hospital. Can you tell me more about that?" Instead of being angry and responding reflexively, Dr Smith changed her approach, which allowed for a good conversation that included an explanation of why Dr Smith was having the student do physical examinations (because the abnormal cannot be recognized until you feel very confident with normal), how the student could better ask questions if she was unsure about Dr Smith's motives, and how Dr Smith could handle her frustrations more appropriately. Putting these strategies into practice increases the ability to get into the space between stimulus and response, so behavior can be directed positively with intention.

Assignments: (1) download 1 of these 2 apps: Breathing Zone or Paced Breathing; practice using the app for at least 10 days to utilize the breath to get into the space; and (2) do at least 1 thing each day that is out of the comfort zone, to practice getting comfortable being uncomfortable. Ideas: start a conversation with a complete stranger, preferably someone in a different generation than you. Take a cold shower in the morning. Eat something you would not normally eat. Sign up for a class doing something you have never done before. Listen to a genre a music that kids or nieces/nephews love but you do not like. Volunteer in an elementary school/middle school/high school or senior living community.

Step 3: Learn How to Speak Other Generational Languages (Social Awareness)

In veterinary medicine, a theme that comes up often when discussing generational conflict is the idea of respect or actually lack of respect. Although it often is the older generation complaining of lack of respect from the younger generations, it increasingly also is heard from the younger generation with regard to the older. This was apparent in the interaction between Dr Smith and her student. Neither of them felt respected. Work done by Jennifer Deal and her colleagues at the Center for Creative Leadership on the issue of respect among generations found that all generations want and value respect.[26] Seemingly, then, this value should not be a point of contention among different generations. Deal's research, however, also discovered that though all generations value respect, the definition of respect differs among generations. In other words, the way each generation "speaks" respect is different. Older generations "want younger people to hold them in higher esteem (than they do others) and to defer to their perspectives," whereas younger generations "want to be held in esteem and to have their opinions considered." Herein lies the problem: we are often not speaking the same language. The solution, in part, comes from suspending bias and from learning another language. For the traditionalist or baby boomer, fielding millennial questions or considering an Xer's opinion is a way to show respect and thereby earn the younger generation's respect. For the Xer or millennial, deferring to wisdom and experience may be an important part of the learning curve that shows respect and allows respect to be earned. Dr Smith could have spoken in the student's language by explaining why she was having her do physical examinations in the first place, not because she did not think the student was capable but because she wanted to the student to better understand normal. The student could have deferred to her older supervisor, trusting that she knew what she was doing from a teaching standpoint.

Sometimes it is an actual language issue that causes problems. Consider the following text exchange between Dr Charles and one of her Generation Z employees.

This is an example of multiple factors that must be taken into account in a multigenerational workplace: method of communication (in-person vs phone vs e-mail vs text), words used in those communication methods, and being willing to learn and grow even if it seems silly or challenging.

Employee: I am going to be a little late because there was an accident on the freeway and I am stuck in some traffic.

Boss: K.

A slight pause and then employee: Are you upset with me?

Boss: No. Why would I be upset? You just did a great job telling me why you were going to be a little late.

Employee: Because you just typed K.

Boss: Isn't that what I am supposed to type? Isn't that just short for OK?

Employee: Ummm…No. I'll explain when I get to work.

When the employee arrived at work, he explained that "K" is not really used as an abbreviation for OK. It typically is used when a significant other is mad or upset and wants to communicate that to his/her significant other. When the author typed K, as her response to the employee's "I'm going to be late" text, he immediately thought she was upset with him. Had the employee not asked the question, it could have led to tension and misunderstanding.

Assignment: watch these videos: https://www.youtube.com/watch?v=WGvC65 GEtuY and https://www.youtube.com/watch?v=2t2Vq834pAA. These are 2 lighthearted examples of how older and younger generations do not always speak the same language.

Step 4: Build Relationships Across Generations (Relationship Management)

Building relationship in the technology-savvy twenty-first century across multiple generations is extremely challenging for 2 main reasons. First, the pace of change in an information age has created a culture of busyness among all generations. Multitasking coupled with the inability to get away from e-mail and work responsibilities thanks to smartphones and wearable technology has diminished the time available to be present and build meaningful professional relationships. Busyness has been embraced as a badge of honor instead of the power of intentional presence.[27] The problem with busyness and multitasking is they are in direct opposition to the skills necessary to build rapport. Second, the younger generations have spent much more time in a virtual world and less time developing face-to-face interpersonal skills.[6,28] If all the generations are to work together effectively, making the time to find common ground and build relationship is a must. This is where a specific skill set within the world of executive coaches (use an ask instead of tell approach to relationship) is really helpful—the art of asking good questions.

Deal's research found that all generations want to learn and almost everyone wants a coach.[29,30] Thus, developing a coaching mindset, whether millennial or baby boomer, Generation X or Generation Z, is a critical skill set for effective generational communication. In his book, *The Coaching Habit*, Michael Bungay Stanier outlines 7 questions that are extremely effective relationship builders because they are built on a coaching foundation. They are (1) What's on your mind? (2) And what else? (3) What's the real challenge here for you? (4) What do you want? (5) How can I help? (6) If you're saying yes to this, what are you saying no to? and (7) What was most useful to you?[31]

Using these questions when you are in the space between stimulus and response, instead of reacting based on emotions, builds rapport and trust. How might the original story have turned out differently if Dr Smith had opted to ask a question instead of barking an order to her student? Upon finishing giving her instructions and listening to Sarah's response, Dr Smith could have recognized she was upset because she felt the student's response was disrespectful, suspended her bias that all millennials are disrespectful because she knows how to speak her student's language (sighing and eye rolling can be an indication of not understanding the motive behind the request- the millennials and Generation Z have been raised to question everything),[14] and said something like, "You seem frustrated about having to do physical exams on the horse's in the clinic. What's on your mind?" That opens the door for the student to share that she is confused about why she has to do physical examinations on basically healthy horses. Dr Smith then can clear up her confusion by explaining the reason she has set the externship up that way. A conversation about how to ask a question when you are confused could also take place once a little trust and rapport has been built.

Assignment: asking good questions take practice. Come up with 5 additional questions to in conversation with someone who is not a member of the same generation in order to build relationship.

SUMMARY

Creating a successful, generationally diverse team requires mindful attention to which strategies build bridges between people and which strategies widen the generation gap. Incorporating emotional intelligence theory into a generational communication strategy that includes recognizing bias, suspending that bias, learning to speak others' languages, and building relationships fosters engagement among all team members and allows generational strengths and abilities to shine.

DISCLOSURE

No commercial or financial conflicts of interest.

REFERENCES

1. Aristotle. Rhetoric. 350BCE. Available at: http://classics.mit.edu/Aristotle/rhetoric.1.i.html. Accessed March 05, 2021.

2. Wen Z, Jaska P, Brown R, et al. Selecting communication media in a multi-generational workplace. Ijbpa; 2010. Available at: https://d1wqtxts1xzle7.cloudfront.net/16689279/generation_x_y_paper__conference_proceeding_draft_2010_1_21.pdf?1339101963=&response-content-disposition=inline%3B+filename%3DSELECTING_COMMUNICATION_MEDIA_IN_A_MULTI.pdf&Expires=1615189187&Signature=ScxitEA~SQegOLocEsWWe09iRLMFG4p1jJbJShZkRL~5u~ZtTfFQO1suW0uNsHacHicRDAn4rZ5Vm11RXO99KmIk0ioTTL6Y60Ir9JhMIETyzftY3gvW3p99JAdXLmautomQL5ifgChhAmqyh2rvV9tXwXNLE0bHO1T56zvx-sS9ws88Ugqz-1n~MiGtN4veU4VgHgCBp60mzT3xEsrIDSBTSuGuLAt1jKzHnAJKpcFyU9EXIZG6XSIbKHoO5k1I5~b2kdyUmSdwRMY38p793qNY6mnQe7SMs-JP6PIq4U56HgeYpDEh27a2sgAETpKg4Fk2ZqH744wGdTSV2p0Mtg__&-Key-Pair-Id=APKAJLOHF5GGSLRBV4ZA. Accessed March 07, 2021.

3. Pew Research Center. The whys and hows of generations research 2015. Available at: https://www.pewresearch.org/politics/2015/09/03/the-whys-and-hows-of-generations-research/. Accessed March 07, 2021.

4. Center for Generational Studies. Hey Dude! Managing age diversity in today's workplace 2007.

5. Tolbize A. Generational differences in the workplace. In: Research and training center on community living. 2008. Available at: http://dwashingtonllc.com/pdf/generational_differences_workplace.pdf. Accessed March 07, 2021.

6. Smyrl BJ. Leading a multi-generational workforce: understanding generational differences for effective communication. In: Marquette university college of professional studies professional Projects. 2011. Available at: https://epublications.marquette.edu/cgi/viewcontent.cgi?article=1029&context=cps_professional. Accessed March 09, 2021.

7. Espinoza C, Ukleja M, Rusch C. The millennials and you, . Managing the millennials. Hoboken: Wiley; 2010. p. 3–12.

8. Deal JJ. Retiring the generation gap: how employees young and old can find common ground. San Francisco: John Wiley & Sons; 2007. p. 5–7, 31–50.

9. Espinoza C, Ukleja M, Rusch C. Managing the millennials: discover the core competencies for managing today's workforce. New Jersey: John Wiley & Sons; 2010. p. 3–11.

10. Center for Generational Studies. Examining a generation's outlook on life 2005.

11. Twenge JA. You can be anything you want to be. In: Generation me: why today's young Americans are more confident, assertive, entitled- and more miserable than ever before. New York: Simon & Schuster; 2006. p. 72–103.

12. Dimock M. Defining generations: where millennials end and generation Z begins. In: Facttank news in the numbers. 2019. Availble at: https://www.pewresearch.org/fact-tank/2019/01/17/where-millennials-end-and-generation-z-begins/. Accessed March 07, 2021.

13. Elmore T. Adjusting the sails: a closer look at generation iY. In: Generation iY: our last chance to save their future. Atlanta: Poet Gardner; 2010. p. 17–28.

14. Twenge JM. You don't need their approval- the decline of social rules. In: Generation me: why today's young americans are more confident, assertive, entitled and more miserable than every before. New York: Free Press; 2006. p. 17–43.

15. Wolford BN. An exploration of generational communication and its impact on military leadership. Greensboro (NC): North Carolina A&T State University Leadership Studies and Adult Education; 2020.

16. Salovey P, Mayer JD. Emotional Intelligence. Imagination Cogn Personal 1990;9:185–211.

17. Goleman D. What makes a leader? Harv Bus Rev 2004;84:1–10.

18. Bradberry T, Greaves J. What emotional intelligence looks like: understanding the four skills. In: Emotional intelligence 2.0. San Diego: Talentsmart; 2009. p. 23–50.

19. Pollack L. Becoming conscious of unconscious bias in the multigenerational workplace. Lindseypollack.com. Available at: https://lindseypollak.com/unconscious-bias-multigenerational-workplace/. Accessed March 09, 2021.

20. Marshall S, Paterson L. Hello brain!. In: The brave athlete: calm the f*ck down and rise to the occasion. Boulder: Velopress; 2017. p. 3–24.

21. Collier A. To better manage millennials check your biases. The Center for Association Leadership. Available at: https://www.asaecenter.org/association-careerhq/career/articles/talent-management/to-better-manage-millennials-check-your-biases. Accessed March 09, 2021.

22. Marshall S, Paterson L. I need to harden the f*ck up, . The brave athlete: calm the f*ck down and rise to the occasion. Boulder: Velopress; 2017. p. 245–58.

23. Nestor J. Exhale. In: Breath. New York: Riverhead; 2020. p. 53–68.

24. Marshall S, Paterson L. I don't like leaving my comfort zone. In: The brave athlete: calm the f*ck down and rise to the occasion. Boulder: Velopress; 2017. p. 215–30.

25. Meyer C. 5 ways to increase your curiosity. In: Atomic object blog. 2013. Available at: https://spin.atomicobject.com/2013/07/18/increase-curiosity/. Accessed March 09, 2021.

26. Deal J. All generations have similar values; they just express them differently. In: Retiring the generation gap: how employees young and old can find common ground. San Francisco: Jossey-Bass; 2007. p. 14–31.

27. Weiland J. Do you wear your busyness like a badge of honor?. In: Mind café. 2020. Available at: https://medium.com/mind-cafe/do-you-wear-your-busyness-like-a-badge-of-honor-777838ece49. Accessed March 09, 2021.

28. Twenge JM. Who is iGen and how do we know?. In: iGen: why today's super-connected kids are growing up less rebellious, more tolerant, less happy and completely unprepared for adulthood. New York: Atria; 2017. p. 1–16.

29. Deal J. Everyone wants to learn- more than just about everything else. In: Retiring the generation gap: how employees young and old can find common ground. San Francisco: Jossey-Bass; 2007. p. 172–93.

30. Deal J. Almost everyone wants a coach. In: Retiring the generation gap: how employees young and old can find common ground. San Francisco: Jossey-Bass; 2007. p. 194–209.

31. Stanier MB. The coaching habit: say less, ask more and change the way you lead forever. Toronto: Box of Crayons Press; 2016.

Challenges in Intercultural Communication

Kelly Farnsworth, DVM, MS, Dipl ACVS*

KEYWORDS

- Nonverbal • Bias • Culture • Stereotype • Cultural competence

KEY POINTS

- Cross-cultural communication is challenging.
- Development of cultural competence is an important process as society becomes more culturally diverse.
- Communication across cultures where language barriers exist requires development of a new set of communication skills.

With the increasing diversity of our clients or potential clients it is important for us as veterinary professionals to recognize the opportunities this affords us to serve a larger demographic. However, along with this opportunity comes the challenges of serving clients for whom English may be a second language as well as clients who may have very different understanding of health care options for their animal. By seeking to become more culturally aware, both as individuals and practices we can have significant impact on the care of our patients. This article focuses on both awareness and skills to aid this process.

CHALLENGES IN INTERCULTURAL COMMUNICATION

The fish only knows that it lives in the water after it is already on the riverbank. Without our awareness of another world out there, it would never occur to us to change.

Unknown

INTRODUCTION

Communication in a veterinary practice setting can be challenging. Add to this the increasing diversity of our clients or potential clients including a significant number of clients who have been raised in different cultures and may speak English as a

Clinical Associate Professor in Equine Surgery, Department of Veterinary Clinical Sciences, Washington State University, 8002 Dry Creek Road, Pullman, WA 99130, USA
* Corresponding author.
E-mail address: Farns005@wsu.edu

Vet Clin Small Anim 51 (2021) 999–1008
https://doi.org/10.1016/j.cvsm.2021.04.017
0195-5616/21/© 2021 Elsevier Inc. All rights reserved.

second language. In the following sections we discuss intercultural competence and nonverbal communication related to different cultures and outline some strategies for dealing with these challenges.

Among health care services, veterinary medicine is distinguished in 2 ways, first by the diversity of its patients and secondly by lack of diversity in veterinary medical providers. Veterinarians and their team members serve not one species but many species and many breeds within each species, whereas from a racial and ethnic standpoint, the veterinary profession is one of the most monolithic in the United States.[1] As the US population continues to become more diverse, Veterinarians increasingly find themselves working with clients who come from a variety of cultures and who hold different worldviews, increasing the need for cultural awareness and competence.[2]

In recent years the AVMA Council on Education has recognized this challenge, and 2017 revised accreditation standards to include as one of the core competencies for graduating veterinarians, diversity, and multicultural awareness, specifically: "Veterinarians demonstrate an understanding of the manner in which culture and belief systems impact delivery of veterinary medical care while recognizing and appropriately addressing biases in themselves, in others, and in the process of veterinary medical care delivery."[3] In addition, the AVMA has developed resources on their Web site to help practitioners better understand cultural competence.

Cultural Competence refers to the ability to interact effectively with people of different cultures.[4] Cultural competence involves 4 components:

- Awareness of one's own cultural worldview
- Attitude toward cultural differences
- Knowledge of different practices and cultural views
- Cross-cultural skills

WHAT IS CULTURE?

Following is a good working definition: culture is the learned and shared knowledge that specific groups use to generate their behavior and interpret their experience of the world.[5] It comprises beliefs about reality, how people should interact with each other, what they "know" about the world, and how they should respond to the social and material environments in which they find themselves. It is reflected in their religions, morals, customs, and the role of animals in their lives (ie, whether they are viewed as property, working animals, or family members). In a veterinary clinical setting, it affects how our clients understand health care, illness, and death associated with their animals. One way to think about culture is to think of it as the "software" of the mind. Essentially, individuals are "programmed" by their cultural group to interpret and evaluate behaviors, ideas, relationships, and other people in specific ways that are unique to their group.[5] Culture is in large part an unspoken, nonverbal phenomenon with most aspects of one's culture being learned though observation and imitation rather than by explicit verbal instructions or expression.[6] Although many facets of culture are internal and invisible, culture is often reflected outwardly in such things as how people behave, how they dress, and the values and ideas they express.

Social scientists often refer to a group of people who share a culture an ethnic group. An ethnic group is a group socially distinguished or set apart by others or by itself, primarily based on cultural or national-origin characteristics.[7] However, it is important to remember that most sizable nations include more than one ethnic/cultural group, and cultural groups are not the same as *racial groups*. Race is a social construct used by scientists and the general public to identify groups of people by physiologic characteristics such as skin color, hair texture, facial features, bone structure, and the like.[7] Most races are made up of many cultures and ethnic groups. Ethnic groups contain *subcultures*, revolving around such things as gender, age, class, race, religion, occupation, or sexual orientation and identity.

In America defining specific cultures can be challenging, as the melting pot has blurred many cultural lines through the process of acculturalization. For example, a Vietnamese immigrant to the United States will most likely retain core cultural values from her native cultural upbringing. These will be added to and modified over time depending on her interactions with the larger US society. Her son or daughter will most likely retain some of the parental values and ideations but will also acquire cultural concepts prevalent in mainstream US society. Her grandchildren, raised by US-born parents and schooled entirely in the United States, may assimilate into the larger society by marrying a non-Vietnamese and adopting a non-Vietnamese lifestyle. This paper is not intended to pigeonhole people into groups, nor should it be interpreted to insinuate that all individuals of any ethnic or cultural group will behave or react in any specific way. The intent of this paper is to simply raise awareness of the challenges faced in a practice setting when dealing with individuals who may come from different cultural backgrounds. In our attempts to become culturally competent we must avoid stereotypes and easy assumptions when delivering health services to different ethnic or cultural groups.

UNDERSTANDING BIAS

As human beings raised on this planet, each of us were raised in or as part of a culture. As previously described, that culture forms what we "know" about the world and how we respond to the social and material environments in which we find ourselves. It is reflected in our religions, morals, and customs. As part of this culture each of us also developed some bias. What is bias? Bias has been defined as a natural inclination for or against an idea, object, group, or individual.[8] Some biases are positive and helpful—as choosing to only eat certain foods or staying away from things that will actively harm us. However, not all bias is healthy. Starting at a young age, no matter what culture or ethnic group we belong to we begin to discriminate between those who are like us, our "ingroup," and those who are not like us, "our outgroup." On the plus side, we can gain a sense of identity and safety. However, taken to the extreme, this categorization can foster an "us-versus-them" mentality, leading to prejudice (preconceived opinion that is not based on reason or actual experience).[8] It is critical that we recognize and learn to control the human tendency to translate "different from me" into "less than me." This unconscious or implicit bias becomes problematic when it causes an individual or a group to treat others poorly as a result of their gender, ethnicity, race, or other factors.[8] The reality is that people are naturally biased, but it does not preclude us from rising higher than our bias.

As part of developing some level of cultural competence we must recognize that each of us have our own implicit bias and that it may be affecting our ability to relate to others in a meaningful way. Implicit or unconscious bias operates outside of an individual's awareness and can be in direct contradiction to a person's espoused beliefs and values. The danger of implicit bias is that it can seep into our affect or behavior without us even being aware of it. Implicit bias toward a certain breed of animal or a certain culture of person can interfere with our clinical assessment, decision-making, and relationship with the client such that the health goals compromised.[9] *Cultural humility* starts with an examination of one's own beliefs and cultural identities and continues as a lifelong process of self-reflection and self-critique.[4] It is not always a comfortable process to turn the microscope inward for first self-evaluation.

STRATEGIES TO IMPLEMENT CULTURAL COMPETENCE

So, what would developing a strategy for cultural competence look like in a veterinary practice? First, as veterinarians we need to apply the diagnostic skills developed through our years of practice to determine where we are as individuals and practices on our journey to cultural competence. As a practice, a starting point might be to start with the AVMA Cultural Competence Self-Assessment Checklist.[10] This online resource will help individuals and practices to identify strengths as well as areas for growth related to cultural awareness. Next, a practice could move to examining the demographics of the practice area to help identify people and animals in the community that might be better served and asking, "are these groups currently be served at a consistently high level?" If the answer is no, then what barriers exist that may inhibit clients from receiving optimal care?

As an example, a practice might identify a significant Spanish speaking population within the practice area.

a. Does the practice have anyone who can speak Spanish?
b. Does the practice have educational materials written in Spanish?
c. Is any of the signage written in Spanish?
d. What do we know about this group of Spanish-speaking individuals?
   1. Are most of the clients or potential clients from one region of the world?
   2. What do we know about that region that might help us better relate to and serve this clientele?

As practice what can we do to educate and raise awareness among our team toward the goal of developing cultural competence? Some of this could be based around learning about the specific cultural groups within the practice area and bringing in a guest speaker to introduce our team to unique aspects of the culture we may not be aware of and help break down stereotypes. It could include utilization of local or online resources to educate the individuals in the practice about implicit bias and how it may be undermining our goals for diversity and inclusion[10] and helping each individual on the team, to ask the hard question, "do I harbor any implicit bias that might be effecting my ability to serve these clients?"

SIX CROSS-CULTURAL COMMUNICATION CHALLENGES
Assumption of Similarity

Many of us naively assume that "people are people" and as such we will all respond similarly in different situations.[11] Although it is true that people around the world share the same basic needs for food, shelter, and security, our attitude surrounding them varies vastly from culture to culture. The assumption of similarity often interferes with our ability to decoding nonverbal signs and signals.[11] Just as there is not one universal spoken language, there also does not seem to be one universal nonverbal language, although emotional expressions are generally recognizable across culture.[12] A person's cultural upbringing will influence to what degree emotions will be displayed or suppressed and to some degree the situations that may bring up emotions. We also need to guard against the reverse assumption that just because someone looks or dresses different than we do, they will automatically have different values and emotions related to their pet care. Most of us have never been trained to look below the surface, beyond language, traditions, and customs, and for differences and similarities that are not immediately obvious. The first step to becoming an effective communicator across cultures is to know what you do not know and look a little deeper for the differences and similarities. When we take the time to learn about those differences and similarities, we open the door to developing mutually beneficial relationships with clients from different cultures.

Language Difference

We have all been introduced to the concept of active listening and effective communication, both verbal and nonverbal. Countless books and educational courses present the same basic message: listen andfocus on the speaker, ask open-ended questions, avoid interruptions, be empathetic, act interested, and make eye contact. You should demonstrate openness and interest with your body language. However, interacting with people from other cultures requires an expanded set of tools.[13]

First, we need to recognize that the communication challenge could be the result of either a language barrier or cultural differences. Communicating with someone new to the English language requires more than talking loudly and slowly and exaggerating our facial expressions. Although as someone who has learned a second language I do appreciate when the person I am talking with slows down and enunciates clearly. The simplest answer to this challenge might be to either learn a second language or hire associate veterinarians and team members who are fluent in the language of target populations in your community. However, we all know this may not be feasible and only addresses the language barrier and not the associated cultural barriers.

The first step in this process is a willingness on our part to engage. As Stephen Covey said in his book Seven Habits of Highly Effective People, "Seek first to understand, then to be understood." In other words, be open to differences and look for similarities. Treat other people with dignity and patience and remember you have a common goal, the health and well-being of the patient.[13] The following 10 steps are adapted from an article written by communications expert Sunita Sehmi.[12,13]

Be empathetic

Put yourself in a nonnative English speaker's shoes. Can you imagine trying to understand a complex disease process explained to you in a second language? We struggle to help many native speakers with these concepts. Add to that situation they may be emotionally charged either due to the severity of disease or the financial challenges associated with treatment. Or imagine the challenge your client has in conveying your message to her family! It is hard enough for us to be effective communicators in our own language. Now imagine conveying medical concepts in a foreign language you are just learning. Empathy is a universal concept.

Be genuinely interested in the client

Focus your attention not only on the message you are delivering but also on what your client is hearing both verbally and none verbally. Make every effort to tailor your communication choices specifically to your listener and be creative. Recognize that just because the client is nodding that may not reflect understanding.

Be patient

Respect and tolerance go a long way in establishing relationships. For some clients, English might not be their native language. Be sensitive to their potential discomfort at not being able to communicate with you. Slow down! Not just in your speech pattern but in the entire encounter. Allow time for individuals in the group to have input with you and with each other. Often one may need to help translate or explain to the other. It is no different than an elderly couple in whom hearing may be compromised.

Focus on similarities to build a common ground
Chances are you have struggled to understand another language. Let your communication partner know you understand that operating in a foreign language is not easy.

Be straightforward and clear
Adjust your medical terminology to the level of the clients understanding. Speak clearly and avoid metaphors, medical jargon, abbreviations, and slang. Be careful, as even humor can easily be lost or misinterpreted; this can be challenging and often requires a bit of probing in the conversation to assess understanding.

Be informed
As discussed earlier, learning about the cultures you serve will help you establish relationships with your clientele. Do not be afraid to ask them about where they are from and what they do for a living. This will help you see them as individuals. Recognize that not all Latin, Asian, or Middle Eastern cultures are alike. Attitudes toward superiors, methods for managing conflict, and even basic communication styles vary greatly. Knowing your team and their background allows you to leverage their strengths.

Mirror your listener
The need to building rapport with clients is critical. Rapport develops into trust, which is essential to good health care. Adapting and matching your communication style with your listeners can be an effective method to bridge cultural gaps we may not understand.

Be aware of and sensitive to all the "cultures" in the room
Remember that there may be multiple cultures and subcultures at play related to ethnicity, gender, age etc. Allow each of them a voice when appropriate. Do not let your personal discomfort dissuade from exploring these cultures and subcultures.

Find and focus on common ground
Do not emphasize differences. When you focus on common goals it becomes easier to reduce the potentially negative impact of differences. As an example, in some cultures the castration of male dogs is frowned on, as it reduces the dog's masculinity. In these cases, focusing on the dog's health and well-being may be more effective than discussing population control.

Use lots of pauses, allowing for clarification and questions and answers
Do not rush. Remember, no one likes to look stupid, and people may need time to process what you say. They may also need time to formulate a response. Although as English-speaking Americans we may be uncomfortable with silence, silence means you are listening. Always ask "what questions do you have?" Assessing understanding is critical. Recognize that when asked "do you understand?" a nod or a yes may not really mean yes. Again no one likes to look stupid. Delivering information in bite size pieces with frequent assessment for understanding builds rapport and increases comprehension.

Nonverbal misinterpretation
As stated earlier just like there is no universal verbal language, there is also not a clear nonverbal language either. Many nonverbal clues or signals share some common origins, and although not exactly the same they can generally be interpreted relatively accurately. However, there are many examples where differences exist.[6] This section does not go into an extensive list of differences but lists a few just for context:

1. Gestures differ dramatically across cultures in meaning, extensiveness, and intensity. Stories abound in the intercultural literature of gestures that signal endearment or warmth in one culture but may be obscene or insulting in another.
2. Eye contact in North America and Western Europe communicates interest and respect, whereas in some Asian cultures looking away from another's eyes almost completely is polite.
3. Personal space and distance vary greatly among different cultures. People from Mediterranean and Latin cultures maintain close distance and may hold hands regardless of gender while talking, whereas Northern European and Northeast Asian cultures maintain greater distance.

So, if we are having a difficult time with verbal communication and now we assert that nonverbal communication may be flawed, the tendency might be to throw our arms in the air and give up. However, it is important for us to remember 2 things:

1. All communication is a 2-way street.
2. Although we may not flawlessly interpret another's nonverbal cues, we are also communicating nonverbally with them. Expressions of warmth, caring, and concern through our nonverbal projection are well received and open further channels.

In addition, as we begin to understand the culture of our clients, we can quickly learn their nonverbal language.

Five Suggestions for Learning the Nonverbal Language of a New Culture

1. As you observe and identify nonverbal cues, remember that your interpretations may not match the intentions of those using the nonverbal cue.
2. Go deeper into the meaning of the nonverbal cue. Many intended meanings do not match superficial explanations, and when you feel there is an incongruency, ask. Check in with the client.
3. Focus on *how* someone says something rather than *what* someone says. Cues in voice, or paralanguage, can lend great insight toward how a person feels toward what they are talking about.
4. Be sensitive to the appropriate nonverbal display rules in a particular situation and cultural community. A simple example of this would be in western/cowboy culture men do not cry in public, which should not be interpreted as them not having feelings or caring about their animal.
5. Learn to decrease your judgmental tendencies and focus more on interpreting the nonverbal cues of others that may be unfamiliar to you.

STEREOTYPES

A stereotype is a fixed, overgeneralized belief about a particular group or class of people.[14] By stereotyping we infer that a person has a whole range of characteristics and attitudes that we assume all members of that group have. The use of stereotypes and categorization is a major way in which we simplify our social world, because they reduce the amount of processing (ie, thinking) we must do when we meet a new person.[1] However, although such generalizations about groups of people may be useful when making quick decisions, they may be erroneous when applied to individuals or are based on misinformation.[15] Stereotyping often leads to prejudice attitudes and discrimination.

As we seek to develop cultural competence, work to learn more about any new culture we need to be particularly aware of stereotyping, not only in the information we are processing but in our own generalizations about the culture we are studying. Always remember each culture is made of a large group of individuals. Each of these individuals may share some cultural similarities but will reflect their own individualisms as well.

Tendency to Evaluate

A common reason for cross-cultural misunderstandings is that we tend to interpret others' behaviors, values, and beliefs through the lens of our own culture and approve or disapprove.[11] To overcome this tendency, it is important to "seek first to understand" the other party's culture. This means not only researching the customs and behaviors of different cultures but going beyond that to understand why people follow these customs and exhibit these behaviors in the first place. As practicing veterinarians, the issue of the human–animal bond (or lack thereof) can be particularly frustrating for those not familiar with societal differences. In many cultures within the United States, people tend to treat their pets as they would their human family members. In other ethnic groups within the United States and other countries, however, cultural differences dictate that animals are treated "as animals."[2]

Recognize that understanding another culture does not necessarily mean we will agree with all of the beliefs and behaviors associated with that culture. However, this understanding allows us a platform to work from to develop mutual understanding around concerns for the health and well-being of the patient we are treating. The fact that the animal is in the clinic tells us we have some common ground; we both care about this animal.

HIGH ANXIETY

Communicating with members of our own culture during times of stress and high anxiety can be difficult. Add language barriers, cultural differences, and urgency to the equation, and the challenge increases exponentially. In addition, stress is a force multiplier when it comes to other cross-cultural challenges previously discussed. Universally all humans share a need for security and certainty, and unfortunately in a health care setting neither one of those is guaranteed. When those needs are not met defensive mechanisms are often used. Defense arousal prevents the listener for concentrating on the message. As a person becomes more and more defensive, they become less and less able to perceive accurately the motives, the values, and the emotions of the sender.[11] Feelings of anxiety usually affected both parties in a stressful intercultural dialogue. In a clinical setting the veterinarian may be uncomfortable because she/he cannot maintain the normal flow of the verbal and nonverbal interaction. There may be language and perception barriers. She/he may be having difficulty understanding the reactions from the client. The client may feel strangely vulnerable and helpless to not only completely understand the problem but to cope with urgency of the situation as well. This discomfort could display in multiple ways but could manifest as withdrawal or as anger. In these situations, it is important for us to step back and process the situation rather than pushing ahead. By evaluating the situation and reflecting on what we have learned about this individual and their culture we may be able to reach into our toolbox and improve the situation.

Not all Cross-Cultural Misunderstandings are a Matter of Culture

Recognize that individual personalities as well as the situation also contribute to the communication challenges in veterinary medicine. As an example, if a client behaves aggressively, is this a reflection of his culture or his personality? When we try to understand why a misunderstanding with somebody from another culture happened, we should consider all aspects by asking the following questions:

- Is there a language barrier?
- Could the reason for the misunderstanding be due to cultural differences?
- Was the misunderstanding perhaps influenced by the situation?
- Or could the misunderstanding be due to personality conflicts?

Cross-cultural communication can be a challenge for many reasons. However, these challenges are not insurmountable and can lead to development of very satisfying and enriching relationships. The first step in this process is really acknowledging that an opportunity exists not only to broaden our client base but also to better serve our current clients. The road to cultural competence starts with clinic and self-evaluation and will continue through life as we interact with more and more people from different cultures.

DISCLOSURE

The author has nothing to disclose.

REFERENCES

1. Labor Force Characteristics by Race and Ethnicity. In BLS Reports # 1088, U.S. Bureau of Labor Statistics 2019. Available at: https://www.bls.gov/opub/reports/race-and-ethnicity/2019/pdf/home.pdf. Accessed February 2021.
2. Sturtz R. Cultural competence: how important is it for veterinary practices? In: clinicians brief. 2014. Available at: https://www.cliniciansbrief.com/article/cultural-competence-how-important-it-veterinary-practices. Accessed February 2021.
3. Larkin M. Diversity, inclusion added to accreditation standards. In: JAMVA News. 2017. Available at: https://www.avma.org/javma-news/2017-08-01/diversity-inclusion-added-accreditation-standards. Accessed February 2021.
4. Cultural competence and cultural humility in veterinary medicine. In: AVMA Online Resources. Available at: https://www.avma.org/resources-tools/diversity-and-inclusion-veterinary-medicine/cultural-competence-and-humility. Accessed February 2021.
5. Cultural Awareness In: National Center for Cultural Competence. Georgetown University Center for Child and Human Development, Curricula Enhancement Module Series. 2014. Available at: https://nccc.georgetown.edu/curricula/awareness/C4.html. Accessed February 2021.
6. Andersen P. Basis of cultural differences in nonverbal communication. In: Samovar L, Porter R, McDaniel E, editors. Intercultural communication: a reader. 13th ed. Boston, MA: Wadsworth Cengage Learning; 2006. p. 294–7.
7. Byrd M, Clayton L. Racial and ethnic disparities in healthcare: a background and history institute of medicine. In: Unequal treatment: confronting racial and ethnic disparities in health care. Washington, DC: The National Academies Press; 2003. p. 474.
8. Bias and Stereotyping. In: psychology today. Available at: https://www.psychologytoday.com/us/basics/bias. Accessed February 2021.
9. Blair IV, Ma JE, Lenton AP. Imagining stereotypes away: the moderation of implicit stereotypes through mental imagery. J Pers Soc Psychol 2001;81(5):828–41.
10. Cultural competence checklist In: AVMA online resources. Available at: https://www.avma.org/sites/default/files/2020-08/Diversity-CulturalCompetenceChecklist.pdf. Accessed February 2021.

11. Barna L. Stumbling blocks in intercultural communication. In: Bennett M, editor. Basic concepts of intercultural communication. 2nd edition. Boston, MA: Intercultural Press; 2013.

12. Paul M. Cultivating cross cultural connection in your veterinary practice. In: DVM 360. Available at: https://www.dvm360.com/view/cultivating-cross-cultural-connection-your-veterinary-practice. Accessed February 2021.

13. Sehmi S. 10 Tips for effective communication in English with non-natives. In: Cultural Intelligence Center. 2014. Available at: https://culturalq.com/blog/10-tips-for-effective-communication-in-english-with-non-natives/. Accessed February 2021.

14. Cardwell M. In: Dictionary of psychology. Chicago: Fitzroy Dearborn; 1999.

15. McLeod S. Stereotypes. In: Simply Psychology. 2015. Available at: https://www.simplypsychology.org/katz-braly.html. Accessed February 2021.

Valuing Diversity in the Team

Adesola Odunayo, DVM, MS*, Zenithson Y. Ng, DVM, MS

KEYWORDS

- Diversity • Inclusion • Underrepresented in veterinary medicine • Racial diversity
- Gender diversity

KEY POINTS

- Diversity is a term used to describe individual and group/social differences (eg, life experiences, personality types, race, socioeconomic status, class, and gender).
- Diversity is about creating a culture and practices that recognize, respect, and celebrate those differences.
- Veterinary practices that are diverse serve a diverse clientele, inspire creativity, and foster innovation.
- Diversity should be valued among team members. This involves continuous lifelong learning as individuals and as a team.

INTRODUCTION

Our ability to reach unity in diversity will be the beauty and the test of our civilization.

—*Mahatma Gandhi*

One of the most impactful ways to create a dynamic team is to foster diversity and inclusivity within the workplace. Workplaces have become more heterogenous over the years, as advances in human, women, and civil rights groups over several decades have spurred greater labor force participation by members of historically underrepresented groups.[1] Studies have shown that leveraging diversity has important implications for the promotion of positive organization change through its facilitation of both individual and organization performance.[2–4] Diverse clientele may be more comfortable and feel more welcome working with people in a diverse workplace. When workplace diversity is approached in a way that maximizes inclusion and minimizes resistance, veterinary organizations will find opportunities to create change

The authors have no conflicts of interest to disclose.
Department of Small Animal Clinical Sciences, The University of Tennessee, 2407 River Drive, Knoxville, TN 37996, USA
* Corresponding author.
E-mail address: aodunayo@icloud.com

that fosters the positive human potential of the members of the team as well as for the clients.[2]

DEFINITION OF THE VETERINARY TEAM

> *To create pride and joy in the workplace, all employees have the right to be involved in the planning of work that affects them.*
> —*Ritz Carlton Leadership Training[5]*

The terms, *relationship-centered care*, *patient safety*, and *medical excellence*, all refer to veterinary practice goals that depend on dynamic interactions of members of the veterinary team.[6] The foundation of good medicine is dependent on the team; thus, it is important to highlight a common definition of what the veterinary team is, for the purpose of this article.[6] There is much variability, however, in how a health care team is defined, both in human medicine and veterinary medicine. Teamwork takes place where hierarchical relationships between doctors, veterinary technicians, assistants, and client services are maintained, together with division of labor flexibility and technical autonomy with interdependence.[7] The authors' approach to the concept of the veterinary team is that it requires every single employee working together to meet the goals of the veterinary practice.

The concept of teamwork varies between work groups. Work groups are composed of individuals responsible for portions of an overall process.[6,8] In the work group model, each practice team member is assigned a specific role and has specific boundaries on what they can or cannot do.[6] Research has shown, however, that work groups have higher numbers of medical errors, lower client compliance, and lower job satisfaction.[6,8] True teams share accountability for outcomes and take full responsibility for the final product.[6,8] They are flexible, synergistic, and ensure quality throughout their job.[6]

Studies in human health care show that positive team environments enhance job satisfaction, provide better role clarity for employees, reduce hospitalization time and cost, improve patient satisfaction and, promote greater team innovation.[9–12] Team care leads to better clinical outcomes and patient satisfaction across human health care settings than does poorly or uncoordinated sequential care.[13]

VETERINARY TEAMS IN PRACTICE

In a standard veterinary practice, whether general or specialty practice, the members of the veterinary team include but are not limited to veterinarians, veterinary technicians, veterinary assistants, management, client-service workers, janitorial staff, and kennel staff. Every team member has a specific role and responsibility toward meeting the goals of the practice; however, team members are synergistic in their roles and are flexible when needed for the common good of the practice. For instance, a kennel staff team worker jumping in to help the front desk check in a client on a particularly busy day demonstrates flexibility and willingness to pitch in to improve the client experience. In an academic institution, members of the team extend to include veterinary students, veterinary technician students, members of the diagnostic laboratories, research staff, and administrative staff. In a research setting, laboratory technicians and postdoctoral scientists join the team with complementary efforts for a dynamic outcome. The focus of this article portrays how diversity affects each and every member of the veterinary team and why diversity should be a priority for team members.

DIVERSITY IN THE TEAM

In the locker room, we speak Spanish, Arabic, Creole. There are people from Latin America, Spain, France … It's an advantage for us. We familiarize ourselves with the culture and language of others.
— *Omar Kreim, Montréal Carabins Intercollegiate Football player[14]*

A lot of different flowers make a bouquet.
— *Islamic Proverb*

Diversity simply means different.[15] Diversity is used to describe individual differences (eg, life experiences, learning and working styles, and personality types) and group/social differences (eg, race, socioeconomic status [SES], class, gender, sexual orientation, country of origin, ability, intellectual traditions, and perspectives as well as cultural, political, religious, and other affiliations) that can be engaged to achieve excellence in practice.[15,16]

Although the term, *diversity*, historically has been focused on race or gender, it is important to recognize diversity extends beyond the surface differences in age, gender, language, or race. Diversity requires recognition of many dimensions, including but not limited to, gender, gender identity, sex, SES, cultural background, language, cognitive style, nationality, age, physical abilities, religious and political beliefs, and other forms of differences—both visible and invisible.[17] Most diversity includes traits, such as gender, cultural background, age, and physical abilities—all of which cannot be controlled or changed. No individual should be discriminated against for the qualities that are inherent to them. Instead, an effort should be made to embrace these differences within a team.

Diversity is about creating a culture and practices that recognize, respect, and value individual differences.[15] In a veterinary team, diversity calls for creating a productive environment in which the equally diverse needs of a client can be met in a creative environment.[15] Diversity should not be an initiative or a project, but it should be an ongoing core aim and a core process that guides the culture of every veterinary organization.[15] From these definitions, it is clear that diversity in the team necessitates the acceptance of different unique aspects of individuals within an institution.[15]

Racial/Ethnic Diversity

Race is a socially constructed system of categorizing human beings based on physically observable features, such as skin color, hair color, eye color, facial features, body types, and/or ancestry. Although race has been used to define people for centuries, there is no genetic basis for the classification.[18] The 2019 American Community Survey, organized by the US Census Bureau, officially recognized 6 racial categories, including people of 2 or more races, in a category called "some other race."[19] In addition, individuals may choose to report more than 1 race to indicate their racial mixture. **Fig. 1** highlights the racial distribution in the United States of America.

The term, *ethnicity*, refers to a group of people who share a common cultural background, such as heritage, culture, ancestry, language, dialect, history, identity, or geographic origin. Members of the same ethnic group may come from the same country or live in the same area.[19,20] For example, people who identify their origin as Hispanic, Latino, or Spanish may be of any race.[19,20] In 2004, the Association of American Medical Colleges executive council defined underrepresented in medicine (URM) as "racial and ethnic populations that are underrepresented in the medical profession relative to their numbers in the general population."[21] In 2017, the American

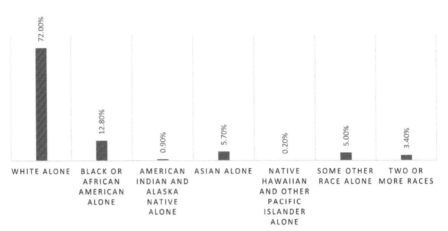

Fig. 1. Population of races in the United States.

Association of Veterinary Medical Colleges (AAVMC) adopted the term, "*underrepresented populations in veterinary medicine*" (*URVM*), for the veterinary profession.[17] On an international level, there may be broad similarities in historically marginalized populations, such as Indigenous and/or First Nations people; however, there also may be continental and country-specific differences in the characterization of underrepresented populations outside of the United States.[17]

Gender and Sexual Orientation Diversity

Understanding gender and sexual orientation diversity begins by understanding some key terms. Biological sex is the genetic material encoded in the chromosome.[22] Gender identity usually is described as an individual's self-defined internal sense of being male or female, regardless of biological sex.[23] It is now recognized, however, that gender identity includes identity between or outside these 2 categories.[23,24] Gender roles are how society expects an individual to behave based on the cultural labels of either being born male or female.[23] Sexual orientation is the predominant erotic thoughts, feelings, and fantasies a person has for a member(s) of a particular sex, both sexes, or neither sex.[23] Individuals who are sexually attracted to the same sex are called homosexual or nonheterosexual, and they make up a minority of adults. Those with predominantly same-sex attraction comprise fewer than 5% of respondents in most surveys.[25] Common terms used in gender and sexual orientation are highlighted in **Table 1**.[26,27]

Sexual orientation is an important fundamental trait that has been understudied and is politically controversial. Although the political rights of lesbian, gay, and bisexual individuals have dramatically improved in Western countries over the past 50 years (including the Marriage Equality Act of 2015), there still is a lot of discrimination geared toward homosexual individuals.[25] For heteronormative individuals growing up in a binary-gendered society, gender identity as male or female is wrongly assumed to be consistent with an opposite-sex sexual orientation and a straight sexual identity. It is important to emphasize that biological sex, gender identity, and gender role do not necessarily bear a relationship to sexual orientation in any individual.[22] Variation on these parameters (eg, cross-dressing or fetishism) also is not linked specifically to sexual orientation.[22]

Table 1
Terms commonly used related to sexuality and gender[26,27]

Commonly Used Terms Related to Gender and Sexual Orientation	Commonly Accepted Meaning
Agender	A person who is not sexually attracted to any gender
Ally	An individual who advocates for and supports members of a community other than their own
Asexual	Having no evident sex or sex organs. May indicate an individual who is not sexually active or sexually attracted to other people
Bias	An inclination or preference that interferes with impartial judgment
Bigendered	An individual whose gender identity is a combination of man and woman
Biphobia	The irrational fear and intolerance of people who are bisexual
Birth sex	The sex one is assigned at birth due to the presence of whatever external sex organs are present
Bisexual, also bi	A person who is attracted to 2 sexes or 2 genders but not necessarily simultaneously or equally
Butch	A lesbian-specific gender identity, originating in women's working-class communities. Associated with the rejection of femininity, in presentation as well as being unavailable to men
Cisgender	A term used to describe people who, for the most part, identify as the gender they were assigned at birth
Coming out	To recognize one's sexual orientation, gender identity, or sex identity and to be open about it with one's self or others.
Drag	The act of dressing in gendered clothing as part of a performance. Drag queens perform in highly feminine attire; drag kings perform in highly masculine attire. Drag performance does not indicate sexuality, gender identity, or sex identity.
Family	A colloquial term used to identify other members of the LGBTIQ community members
Gay	Men attracted to men. Colloquially used as an umbrella term to include all LGBTIQ people
Gender	(1) A socially constructed system of classification that ascribes qualities of masculinity and femininity to people. (2) One's sense of self as masculine or feminine regardless of external genitalia. Gender characteristics can change over time and are different between cultures.
Gender conformity	When one's gender identity and sex "match" (ie, fit social norms)
Gender expression	The way one presents oneself to the world, as either masculine or feminine or both or neither

(continued on next page)

Table 1 (continued)	
Commonly Used Terms Related to Gender and Sexual Orientation	**Commonly Accepted Meaning**
Gender fluid	A person whose gender identification changes, whether within or outside of societal, gender-based expectations
Gender identity	An individual's self-awareness or fundamental sense of themselves. The gender that one sees oneself as. This can include refusing to label oneself with a gender.
Gender-neutral	Nondiscriminatory language to describe relationships. *Spouse* or *partner* are gender-neutral alternatives to gender-specific words like *husband* or *wife*.
Gender queer	An individual who redefines or plays with gender or refuses gender altogether
Heterosexuality	Sexual, emotional, or romantic attraction to a sex other than your own. This is commonly thought as "attraction to the opposite sex" but because there are not only 2 sexes, this definition is inaccurate.
Homophobia	The irrational fear and intolerance of people who are homosexual or of homosexual feelings within one's self
Homosexuality	Sexual, emotional, and/or romantic attraction to the same sex
Intersex	A set of medical conditions that feature congenital anomaly of reproductive and sexual system. Intersex individuals are born with "sex chromosomes," external genitalia, or internal reproductive systems that are not considered "standard" for either male or female.
In the closet	Keeping one's sexual orientation and/or gender or sex identity a secret
Invisible minority	A group whose minority status not always is immediately visible, such as some disabled individuals and LGBTIQ individuals
Lesbian	A woman attracted to women
LGBTIQ, LGBTQIA, LGBTQ+	Lesbian, gay, bisexual, transgender, intersex, queer Lesbian, gay, bisexual, transgender, queer, intersex, ally Lesbian, gay, bisexual, transgender, queer. The "+" signifies one may identify with a sexual orientation or gender identity not represented in this acronym (eg, pansexual).
Nonbinary	A term for gender identities that fall outside the gender binary
Oppression	Results from the use of institutional power and privilege where 1 person or group benefits at the expense of another

(continued on next page)

Table 1 (continued)	
Commonly Used Terms Related to Gender and Sexual Orientation	**Commonly Accepted Meaning**
Pansexual	A person who is fluid in sexual orientation and/or gender or sex identity
Polyamory	The practice of having multiple open love relationships
Pre-op	A transsexual who has not yet had their sex change operation but plans on it
Queer	An umbrella term used to refer to all LGBTIA people. It also is a political statement, as well as sexual orientation, which advocates breaking binary thinking and seeing both sexual orientation and gender as potentially fluid. It also can be used as simple label to explain a complex set of sexual behaviors and desires.
Rainbow flag	The internationally recognized official flag of the LGBTIQ civil rights movement
Sexual orientation	The deep-seated direction of one's sexual attraction. It is on a continuum and not a set of absolute categories.
Straight	A person who is attracted to a gender other than their own
Transgender	Individuals whose psychological self differs from the social expectations they were born with. For example, a female with a masculine gender identity. It also is an umbrella term for transsexuals, cross-dressers, gender queers, and people who identify as neither male nor female or as neither a man nor a woman.
Transsexual	An older term for individuals whose gender identity is different from their assigned sex at birth, who seek to transition from male to female or female to male. Many people do not use this term as it sounds overly clinical.

Transgender individuals live with a gender identity that is different from traditional binary gender roles or their birth sex. In essence, the term, *transgender*, reflects the concept of breaking gender roles and gender identity and/or transcending the boundaries of one gender to another gender. Some transgender individuals also are transsexual. This is because transgender individuals may seek genital surgery and can be either pretransition/operative, transitioning/in the process of hormonal and surgical sex reassignment, or post-transition/operative.[23]

Ableism and Visible and Invisible Diversity

The Americans with Disabilities Act (ADA) defines an individual with a disability as a person "who has a physical or mental impairment that substantially limits one or more major life activity," whereas the World Health Organization defines disability as "an umbrella term for impairments, activity limitations and participation restrictions."[28,29] Disabilities may be visible and require assistance devices, such as wheelchairs or blind canes, or they may be invisible, such as depression, autism spectrum disorder, or dyslexia—all of which are mentally impairing. There is a correlation between age and physical disability, indicating that with increasing age comes increasing likelihood of having a physical disability.[30] Irrespective of the details of the particular disability, the ADA prohibits discrimination on the basis of disability in employment, government, public accommodations, commercial facilities, transportation, and telecommunications. Additionally, the decision to disclose a disability is a personal one,[31] so it cannot be asked of the individual if they have a disability or what their disability is. Overall, there is a lack of diversity training focused on disabilities, which contributes to the lack of awareness and comfort working with and including these individuals.[32,33] Proactive leadership in this arena is critical in supporting these individuals in positive ways.[30]

A disability may have an impact on an individual's ability to complete a task, especially in a physically and mentally demanding job in the veterinary workplace. For example, animal restraint and lifting heavy animals may be challenging for someone with a physical impairment, whereas the sound of barking dogs may be overstimulating to a neurodiverse individual. Accommodations must be made to meet the needs of these individuals at work, such as providing appropriate breaks for recovery or doctor's appointments. The employer and staff comply with these accommodations to encourage and permit these individuals to thrive in the workplace.

Although these accommodations may be perceived as a barrier, there are far-reaching benefits of including individuals with disabilities on the team. Acknowledging and assisting an individual to conquer barriers to succeed at their job builds empathy and teamwork. Empathy comes with other employees seeing not only that an individual is seen for their disability and limitations but also that the individual has so many attributes to offer. Additionally, working with an individual with a disability opens others' minds to different ways to accomplishing a task. This facilitates the critical concept that equality and equity are not the same; equality gives everyone the same exact resources whereas equity distributes resources based on the needs of the individual.[34] People with disabilities may not have been afforded the opportunity to showcase their strengths and talents. Allowing a person with a disability to succeed at an unconventional job can be empowering to others living with similar disabilities.[31]

One area that is controversial in terms of disability diversity is the need for an assistance animal in the workplace. Although it is recommended that an individual cannot discriminate against someone for having a service animal, it may be unsafe or prohibited in the veterinary workplace.[35,36] The AAVMC published a set of guidelines regarding service animals in 2019.[37] According to the guidelines, "Legally, service animals are allowed to accompany the individual with a disability in all areas of a medical facility where health care personnel, visitors, and patients are normally allowed during inpatient services unless the animal's presence or behavior creates a fundamental alteration in the nature of a facility's services in a particular area or is a direct threat to other persons in a particular area."[37] Policies governing service animals must balance the benefits a service animal provides for its handler with the risks posted by the service animal to other animals or human beings.[37]

Socioeconomic Diversity

Socioeconomic diversity is achieved by inclusion of individuals of varying SES, which is the social standing or class of an individual typically based on a combination of education, income, and occupation.[38] SES determines where an individual lives, what they eat, what activities they engage in, and with whom they associate. SES also has a complicated relationship with race and health status,[39] which contributes to the expanding discussion on race. Social equity has been challenged due to the income inequalities and larger wage gaps between lower, middle, and upper classes.[40]

There is inherent economic disparity among different occupations within the same workplace; veterinarians, upper-level management, technicians, and support staff each earn different salaries. Salary alone, however, does not designate SES, because other factors, such as supplemental jobs, previous careers, debt, family backgrounds, and spouses, contribute to SES. Thus a critical lesson in diversity and inclusion is that an individual's background never should be assumed. Employers who exclude class from discussions of diversity and inclusion risk missing the opportunity to enhance the talents and success of the organization, because the most diverse workplaces, socio-economically and beyond, tend to be most profitable.[41]

There are numerous benefits from the inclusion of a socioeconomically diverse staff. Socioeconomic diversity contributes to more frequent interactions across class lines, promoting a more positive environment.[42] An individual's SES also may dictate life-styles, such as the type of food eaten and how an individual may spend breaks. Working with individuals from various social classes exposes an individual to a diversity of interests, hobbies, and life perspectives that may spark new ideas for workplace bonding activities for all to enjoy. In addition, an individual from a lower SES may have been limited to exposure and opportunities in veterinary medicine, perhaps due to inability to pay for education or the need to pursue higher wage employment than what the veterinary workplace can afford. These individuals should be encouraged to grow to become social class transitioners.[43] An example of a social class transitioner may be an inexperienced individual starting as a veterinary assistant who is given the tools and opportunities to pursue continuing education to become a veterinary technician and who then demonstrates their skills to climb the leadership ladder to becoming an upper-level manager. Not only does this process allow for the success of the individual, but they prove to be individuals with the credibility to better relate and communicate with various groups and serve as role models for others who can achieve similar paths.

Employees of higher SES who are sensitive and aware of the importance of socio-economic diversity are valuable in the workplace. Although individuals of any class can serve as mentors, more affluent individuals can provide good leadership and guidance to those from economically disadvantaged backgrounds. These leaders with dispensable incomes often have the opportunity to give to their staff members in simple ways, such as treating the team to food, gifts of gratitude, and bonding activities outside of work. Everyone should be sensitive that not every individual may be able to financially afford leisure activities and items that others may enjoy, and engaging in this may inadvertently foster exclusion in the workplace. In addition, a powerful way individuals can promote inclusion and a positive workplace is to contribute to a colleague in need, such as when tragedy strikes. These thoughtful financial and emotional methods of support of team members, regardless of background, can have long-lasting and far-reaching effects on the cohesiveness of the workplace.

Age Diversity

Age is defined as the length of time a person has lived or a thing has existed.[44] The current workplace spans a wide range of ages, including

Traditionalists (born 1925–1945)
Baby boomers (born 1946–1964)
Generation X (born 1965–1980)
Generation Y (millennials) (born 1981–2000)
Generation Z (iGen) (after 2001)[45]

Interactions among individuals in different age grounds in the workplace may create situations that may be exclusive to some. Common stereotypes may include statements that the younger generations are all creative and older team members may struggle with new technology. Age diversity embraces the inclusion of various generational groups in a setting and often is overlooked in discussions of diversity and inclusion but is no less important than the typical characteristics of gender and race.[46] Although challenges in working across generational gaps exist, there are numerous ways to overcome and conquer them, promoting a rich working environment.[47] Furthermore, specific laws prohibit age discrimination, such as the Age Discrimination in Employment Act of 1967, which protects applicants and employees over 40 years of age from discrimination on the basis of age in hiring, promotion, compensation, terms, conditions, or privileges of employment.[48]

Any place of employment that maintains age diversity benefits from a stronger and more productive workplace.[49] This is because of the creativity, invigoration, and motivation that result from working across generations. Traditionally, older generations serve as role models who pass on the lessons that only experience can teach and younger generations lack. An opportunity to teach may be a welcome change by an older individual because it takes the teacher away from the monotony of everyday work tasks. Conversely, younger generations come with fresh and cutting-edge perspectives that can enlighten older generations. Younger generations also have the distinct advantage of being more technologically and social media savvy than older generations. These differences drive innovation through teaching one another different ways of accomplishing the same task. This mutual mentorship is a dynamic relationship of give and take where both parties and the organization at large benefit. Both older and younger colleagues corroborate that age diversity in the workplace increases motivation and intent to stay with an organization.[50] This increased intent to stay not only reduces employee turnover but also improves the stability of an organization by ensuring that these younger individuals are appropriately trained to assume the positions of the older individuals when retirement commences. The young then will serve as old once retirement nears, which promotes stability.

In addition, millennials and Generation Z-ers arguably are the most diverse and inclusive generations. Mixing individuals from these generations will propagate further diversity in the workplace.[51]

The Concept of Intersectionality

The concept of intersectionality emerged as a critique of social movements' tendency to exclude the interest of underrepresented groups and identities.[52] Defined in 1989 by Kimberle Crenshaw, an American lawyer, civil rights advocate, and philosopher, intersectionality describes multiple threat of discrimination when individuals' social identities overlap and contribute to systemic oppression and discrimination.[53–55] It is a framework that promotes an understanding of human beings as shaped by interacting social locations and identities (eg, race, sexuality, gender expression, age, ability, religion, and SES).[53] Crenshaw initially used this term to describe experiences of Black women who experience both sexism and racism.[55] It is the difference in experiences among people with different overlapping identities. For example, a Black, gay, disabled woman faces very different threats of discrimination from a Black, straight, able-bodied woman. The concept of intersectionality is important when attempting to understand and address interwoven prejudices faced by many individuals every day. Being cognizant about the concept of intersectionality helps achieve the goals of celebrating diversity in the workplace. Team members must recognize differences and not assume all members of the same group (eg, women) feel a certain way. Team members should avoid oversimplified languages that might define people by a single identity (eg, a practice manager getting feminine scrubs for female employees, thus assuming all women are defined by their body types).[56] Analyzing the workspace to ensure diversity of all kinds is represented also is helpful. A workplace may be racially and ethnically diverse but may not be accessible to people with disability. It is important to evaluate the work environment constantly for welcoming or distancing practices.[56] Team members should take the time to listen to people with different experiences however should not expect individuals with different identity markers different to want to educate others. It is important team members seek out existing intersectional narratives available to educate themselves.[56]

BENEFITS OF DIVERSITY

We are all different, which is great because we are all unique. Without diversity, life would be very boring.

—*Catherine Pulsifer*

What drives a city's innovation engine, then—and thus its wealth engine—is its multitude of contrasts. The more and greater the contrasts, and the more they are marbled together, the better. The most productive city is one with many cultures, many languages, and more kinds of urban experience available than any citizen can keep track of

—*Stewart Brand*[57]

Diversity and inclusion increasingly are recognized as requirements for optimal team performance because diversity has been proved to improve financial performance, leverage talent, increase innovation, and improve team performance.[58] The case for diversity also includes the ability to serve a diverse group of clients, provide diverse mentors at all levels, bring different points of views to debates and problem solving, better engage the community, and include investigators with a broad range of perspectives in scholarly activities.[58] In addition, underrepresented groups were found more likely to be attracted to organizations with underrepresented employees; thus, diversity ultimately helps increase the talent pool of applicants for a position.[1,59]

In human medicine, increasing URMs in the workforce directly improves health care for medically underserved populations, which ultimately benefits the entire population at large.[60,61] The benefits of diversity are seen in the desire to meaningfully explore areas of differences and commonality in the team in a manner that promotes self-awareness and confronts conscious and unconscious bias in a safe, positive, and inclusive manner.[17] A summary of benefits of diversity in the workplace is highlighted in **Box 1**.

In veterinary medicine, clients have the freedom to choose which veterinary practice they utilize. Although many factors may play into an individual's choice to use 1 practice over another, the impact that the diversity of a clinic has on the decision cannot be denied. For example, a transgender person of color who is a native Spanish speaker may be apprehensive about visiting a clinic where the employees are homogeneously White and English-speaking. Having a Spanish-speaking or transgender person or a person of color on staff with whom this client can relate, communicate, and connect with can be a compelling reason for the individual to choose this clinic. Diverse clientele may be more comfortable and feel more welcome working with people in a diverse workplace. This powerfully illustrates that the clinic is inclusive of all populations, especially in a profession that is not diverse. Therefore, a diverse veterinary team begets diverse veterinary clientele.

Box 1
Summary of the benefits of diversity in a team

Wide range of skill sets

Different viewpoints and better problem solving

Serves a diverse clientele

Good performance and better results

Increased adaptability

Availability of diverse mentors

Inspires creativity and fosters innovation

Great opportunity for personal and professional growth

Increased productivity

Attracts and retains the best talent

Although the overall benefits of diversity are positive, there are a few challenges associated with implementing diversity in the workplace. These include the actual implementation of diversity, communication barriers due to cultural differences, and resistance to change. Practical tips to help overcome some of the challenges posed by having a diverse team are discussed later.

CURRENT STATUS OF DIVERSITY IN VETERINARY MEDICINE

An individual has not started living until he can rise above the narrow confines of his individualistic concerns to the broader concerns of all humanity.
—Martin Luther King, Jr

Embracing diversity is vital if the veterinary profession continues to fulfill its mission of serving all communities and animals.[62,63] Diversity touches all aspects of the profession, from improving communication with clients to providing a better understanding of cultural attitudes and practices that affect animal care.[62] Diversity also provides the veterinary professional an insight into how differences in gender attitudes affect the work environment.

The US Census Bureau estimates that racial/ethnic underrepresented groups make up about a third of the US population, with more than half of all children predicted to be minorities by 2023.[63,64] Ethnic/racial underrepresented groups also are projected to make up 54% of the nation's population by 2050.[63,64] Contrary to societal trends, veterinary medicine remains one of the least racially/ethnically diverse professions in the United States.[63,65,66] The American Veterinary Medical Association (AVMA) estimated that in 2011%, 90% of veterinarians were White.[63] The numbers of URVM strongly indicate that the veterinary profession does not reflect the US population racially. Compared with the US Census Bureau numbers (see **Fig. 1**), approximately 5% of US veterinarians are estimated to be Hispanic, 2% Black, 1% Asian/Pacific Islander, and less than 1% American Indian/Alaskan native.[67] A systemic review published in 2017 identified cultural/language barriers in 24% (12/51) of articles that investigated obstacles to obtaining adequate veterinary care.[68] The fear of not being understood, being taken advantage of, or being judged may discourage clients from seeking the care their pets need.[68]

Much positive change has happened to increase racial/ethnic diversity in veterinary medicine. The AVMA, AAVMC, colleges of veterinary medicine, and various individuals have demonstrated committed effort to increase the population of URVM.[63,67,69] The AAVMC launched the DiVersity Matters initiative in 2005, and enrollment of URVM has increased approximately 134% in colleges of veterinary medicine subsequent to that initiative (**Fig. 2**).[63,66] The AAVMC now reports that approximately 20% of total enrollment in colleges of veterinary medicine are URVM.[63,66,70] This change emphasizes that progress can be made with purposeful commitment to the cause of enhancing diversity. As demonstrated in **Fig. 3**, however, compared with the rest of the general population, there still is much to be done to increase the number of URVM in the profession.

There currently are few data about racial diversity in other members of the veterinary team (veterinary technicians, veterinary assistants, and members of client services), because discussion on diversity tends to focus on veterinarians.[71] Based on the authors' experiences across veterinary institutions over the country, however, team members represented in those roles still largely are White. A study investigating veterinary technician specialist salaries in 2013 reported demographics as part of the study.[72] Of 321 respondents, 336 (95.7%) were female and 14 (4%) were male, with 1 individual not answering the question. Most, 335 (95.4%) identified as White. The racial/ethnic identity of the other respondents was not reported in the article.[72] If enhanced diversity and inclusion in the veterinary is desired, it is important to include all members of the veterinary team.[71]

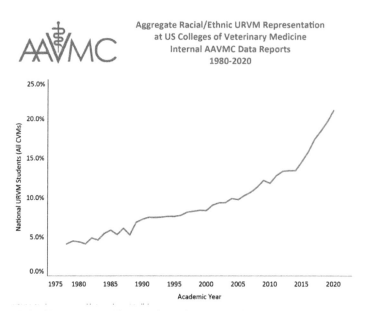

Fig. 2. Graph highlighting enrollment of racial/ethnic underrepresented individuals in veterinary medical colleges from 1975 through 2020. The most significant increase is noted after the DiVersity Matters initiative was started in 2005.[70] Total DVM student enrollment at the US colleges of veterinary medicine is 13,548. (*From* Association of American Veterinary Medical Colleges. Annual Data Report 2019-2020 (Internet). 2020:1-64. http://www.aavmc. org/About-AAVMC/Public-Data.aspx.)

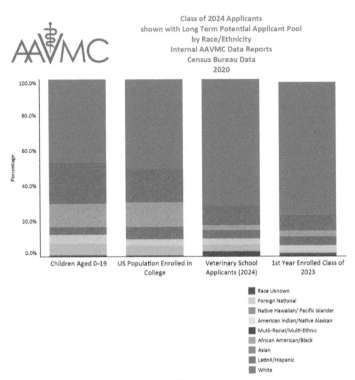

Fig. 3. Bar chart showing representation of different racial groups—children in the general US population, general US population enrolled in college, veterinary school applicants, and the first-year enrolled class of 2023.[70] Census data from the 2017 American Community Survey. The total number of applicants to the class of 2024 was 8152. (*From* Association of American Veterinary Medical Colleges. Annual Data Report 2019-2020 (Internet). 2020:1-64. http://www.aavmc.org/About-AAVMC/Public-Data.aspx.)

Other than the many challenges of veterinary practice (high education debt, stressful work environment, and so forth), URVM also face the additional challenges of discrimination, microaggression, and systemic racism. Systemic racism is a relic of colonialism, capitalism, and slavery.[73] It operates by maintaining, justifying, and, in some cases, encouraging racist behaviors.[73] Research shows that the world still is shaped by systemic racism.[74–77] URVM team members have to worry about themselves, family, and friends being wrongly accused, physical assaulted, or even killed because of racial bias.[73–76] In 2020, the Multicultural Veterinary Medical Association released a video, *Wake Up, Vet Med*, that shares the stories of racism and discrimination experienced by URVM.[78] Systemic racism, discrimination, and microaggressions also contribute to the low racial/ethnic diversity seen in veterinary medicine due to significant barriers that prevent URVM from applying, be accepted to, or succeeding in veterinary school.

When considering gender diversity, the number of female veterinarians in the profession has increased significantly over time. In the nineteenth century, the idea of women as veterinarians violated masculine livestock culture and threatened the professional aspirations of male veterinarians.[79,80] This was evidenced by the following admissions policy at Kansas State University in 1939:

We do not encourage women to enroll in the curriculum in veterinary medicine. In fact, we try to discourage them, our reason being that we must refuse admission to many worthy young men, and to accept a young woman with the chances that she will not remain in the profession and to deny admission to a young man, does not seem logical.[79,81]

In 1970 to 1971, women comprised only approximately 8% of practicing veterinarians.[79] Due to changes in sex discrimination laws, potential loss of federal funding, and an increased demand for veterinary services, veterinary schools across the country started admitting more women into veterinary school.[79] Currently, approximately 80% of veterinary students are women, a significant reversal of proportion.[79] This also is visualized in the 2019 to 2020 AAVMC annual data report (**Fig. 4**). This is a positive change for veterinary medicine, because many other science, technology, engineering, and mathematics professions struggle with poor representation of the female gender. Despite being the majority gender in the profession, however, women still have lower salaries than men, are less likely to own their practices, and work often as associates in practices owned by others.[79,82]

Due to the number of women in veterinary medicine, members of the male and members of the nonbinary gender are URVM based on gender. The AAVMC started collecting information on nonbinary students in 2017, and it is estimated that approximately 0.10% of the professional doctor of veterinary medicine (DVM) student population in the 2019 to 2020 academic year are nonbinary.[70] The authors currently are unaware of specific data on the number of transgendered individuals in veterinary medicine. There is strong social and scientific evidence, however, that nonbinary

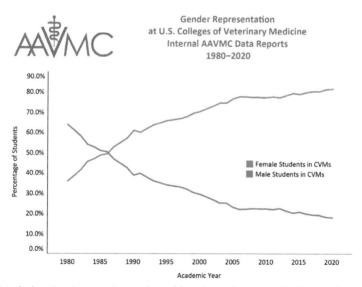

Fig. 4. Graph showing increase in number of female students enrolled in veterinary medical colleges from 1980 to 2020.[70] In 2017, AAVMC began collecting data for individuals identifying as nonbinary. For the 2019–2020 academic year, these individuals comprised 10% of the professional DVM student population. Total enrollment at the US colleges of veterinary medicine is 13,548. (*From* Association of American Veterinary Medical Colleges. Annual Data Report 2019-2020 (Internet). 2020:1-64. http://www.aavmc.org/About-AAVMC/Public-Data.aspx.)

and transgendered individuals are marginalized, harassed, and discriminated against in social settings, the workplace, health care, and academia.[83–86] In addition, nonbinary and transgendered individuals disproportionately experience victimization, physical, and sexual violence compared with male and female individuals.[87–89] The higher incidence of suicide and suicide attempts in this group of individuals is thought to be due to minority stress[90–92]

WHY DO PROPORTIONS MATTER?

Prejudice is a burden that confuses the past, threatens the future and renders the present inaccessible.
—Maya Angelou

It is helpful to highlight some of personal challenges experienced by underrepresented individuals in the workplace. Those challenges may include[78,93,94]

- Feeling the pressure to conform and make fewer mistakes
- Feeling more visible and on display
- Trying to become socially invisible so as not to stand out
- Finding it harder to gain credibility
- Being more isolated and under-respected
- Being more likely to be excluded from informal peer networks
- Having fewer opportunities to be sponsored
- Facing misperceptions about their identity and role in the organization
- Being more likely to be stereotyped
- Facing more personal stress
- Feeling like they did not earn their place (imposter syndrome) and were hired to check boxes as a token (ie, organizations hiring a racial or gender underrepresented individual to fulfill institutional hiring guidelines)
- Feeling underemployed and/or overused by departments or institutions
- Having their authority challenged by students and/or employees
- Having minimal guidance and mentoring towards promotion, tenure and reappointment
- Dealing with colleagues who either ignore them or make racist comments about aspects, such as appearance or accent
- Disparagement of scholarly activity due to a focus on racial or ethnic issues

Veterinary institutions must make changes to increase diversity to reap the positive institutional benefits of a diverse organization. An increase in diversity also has positive benefits for the URVM, by reducing the impact of these aforementioned challenges felt by URVM. The more individuals that share common characteristics, the less isolating and less stressful the work environment is for those individuals.

VALUING DIVERSITY IN THE TEAM

When we listen and celebrate what is both common and different, we become a wiser, more inclusive, and better organization.
—Pat Wadors

Good leadership requires you to surround yourself with people of diverse perspectives who can disagree with you without fear of retaliation.
—Doris Kearns Goodwin

Appreciating and valuing diversity of the veterinary team is an important and intentional task. It also is a lifelong commitment to learning more about the differences in team members while celebrating those differences. It ensures all team members feel included, valued, and welcomed. Valuing diversity also involves standing up for URVM team members when in the majority. The rest of this article focuses on action steps veterinary teams can take to support diversity.

Promote Training in Diversity, Equity, and Inclusion

The first steps to promoting and celebrating diversity are education and knowledge. Gaining awareness of the different types of diversity present among team members, understanding why diversity is important, and learning how to support URVM members of the team. Hospital managers and administrators should provide opportunities for specific training on issues surrounding diversity geared toward the entire veterinary team. This training could include specific certificate programs (like the Certificate for Diversity and Inclusion in Veterinary Medicine by Purdue University),[95] seminars given by experts in the field or having centrally available resources (books and links to Web sites) for the veterinary team.

Making such training mandatory will ensure the entire team is involved in the learning process but it also may create feelings of having to do additional work in some members of the team. Whether training is determined to be mandatory or voluntary, what is most important is that veterinary team leaders are exemplary models in acquiring knowledge as well as demonstrating the ability to lead inclusively and enhance equity in the workplace.[96] Team leaders should realize that their organization is not a level playing field, and actions should be taken to promote equity in the organization. *Fair opportunity* is not the same for everyone and team leaders should express their motivation, as well as barriers, for countering inequality, set goals toward greater equity, and take action.[96] This will signal a commitment to the rest of the team members and these principles will lead to enhancement of diversity and inclusion efforts in the community.[96]

Having leaders committed to enhancing diversity, equity, and inclusion (DEI) as well as promoting training among team leaders also leads to an increase in the number of diverse employees hired on a team because of the development of relationships and respect and trust among team members as well as the institution of best hiring practices.

Standing Together Against Racism

Despite many advances of the post–civil rights era, people of color (POC) still face many obstacles and experience discrimination in their everyday lives in the modern day.[97] POC earn less than Whites at every educational level and remain overrepresented among unskilled workers while still being underrepresented in managerial positions.[76,98–101] Studies have shown that racism very much remains a persistent, if not routine and systemic, feature of work life, thus contributing to the organization of society in ways that structurally disadvantage POC.[76] In addition to racism from employers and colleagues in veterinary institutions, POC often face racism from clients who seek care at veterinary institutions.[73,78] Experiencing or witnessing racism has an impact on POC in several ways, including having a direct impact on their mental, emotional, and psychological well-being as well as having a negative impact on their careers.[76,102] Specific ways veterinary teams can stand together with their POC colleagues include

1. Systemic evaluation of how teams are structured: in a recent large survey of POC and White British employees over 16 years old, a large majority reported that they did not know or were unsure of what their employer did to promote equality, diversity, and fairness.[76] Some employees even suggested that promotion of equality and diversity was "nonexistent."[76] Traditional DEI programs are designed to increase minority representation but usually do not challenge the racial hierarchies that are built in the organization, which may explain the low number of POC in leadership roles. Instead of focusing on how to increase racial diversity in the workplace, veterinary organizations must question why so much power remains with White people.[76,103] Veterinary organizations must be willing to interrogate aspects of their workplace that they currently take for granted and make publicized changes to their infrastructure as it relates to racism.[76,104] This may include implementing accountability metrics for merit-based pay and increasing transparency of decision-making managers.[76,104] Bold actions are needed to disrupt the status quo, as demonstrated by Reddit cofounder Alexis Ohanian, who stepped down from the board of directors and asked for his seat to be replaced with a Black person.[76,105] Systemic racism should be seen beyond individual behaviors to discriminatory procedures, unfair policies, and biased practices that result in inequitable outcomes for URVM.[76]

2. Creating a no tolerance policy: leaders of veterinary teams should create and enhance a no tolerance policy against racism.[106] And although this policy needs to be initiated by the leaders/administration of the organization, every team member needs to take a stand. If a client or team member says something racist (examples may include not wanting a POC team member to provide care or services, making a racist joke or comment, or sharing a social media post that is hateful), other members of the team need to be vocal about their inability to condone that kind of speech or behavior.[107] Clients and team members who threaten a culture of diversity and inclusion should not be allowed to propagate their speech and behavior. Although this framework may seem harsh, it sets a strong and powerful tone to safeguard the inclusion of all members of the community.

3. Creating antiracism resources in organizations: antiracism is taking action directly against racism.[76] McCluney and colleagues[76] suggested utilizing Newton's first law of motion to view antiracism. An entity (ie, racism) remains in motion unless it is compelled to change its state by an opposing external force (ie, antiracism).[76] It is not enough, or perhaps grossly inadequate, for team members to be "not-racist."[76,108] "All policies, ideas, and people are either being racist or antiracist."[108] For instance, a team member may believe carrying out an everyday task is harmless and does not demonstrate racism; however, the ability to carry on business as usual and ignore the everyday microaggressions and injustice affecting Black people and other POC continues the motion of racism and is not antiracist.[76,108] Antiracism includes a continual commitment to learning about racism, acknowledging racist mistakes, and creating equitable structures to replace systems that maintain White supremacy and marginalization of POC.[76,109] Owners, managers, and members of the veterinary administration can create and share antiracism resources in the workplace.[76] Members of the veterinary team also should adopt a long-term view for learning about antiracism and view it as a long journey of reflection, growth, and change.[76]

4. Equal pay for equal work: there is a long history of wage gaps in the workforce of numerous industries that demonstrates inequalities in gender and race.[110] Despite the narrowing of wage gaps in recent years, large racial and gender gaps in the

United States persist. Pay grades should be based on experience and skills without regard to demographics.

Encourage Language that Promotes Inclusion

The fact that language plays a central role in the way human beings behave and think is accepted nearly universally.[111] Inclusive language is defined as words and phrases that reflect and respect the diverse identities in society and in the workplace.[112] The use of inclusive language in organizations increases creativity and promotes DEI efforts.[111,113] In essence, inclusive language is respectful, accurate, and relevant to all. Key drivers of inclusive environments are organization leaders who work to integrate inclusive language into their organization's culture.[112,114]

Inclusive language also changes over time to reflect language that is the least harmful and exclusionary.[112] And even as such phrases continue to evolve, the Linguistic Society of America describes inclusive language as, "Inclusive language acknowledges diversity, conveys respect to all people, is sensitive to differences and promotes equal opportunities."[112,115] Language that is not inclusive can unintentionally marginalize some members of the team.[112] Specific circumstances where inclusive language should be considered are outlined, but it always is a good idea, when in doubt, to ask team members which terms/words they prefer. **Table 2** highlights other words that can be used to promote inclusion in the workplace.[112]

1. POC: there are a few catch-all terms used to refer to racial groups who are not White. Some of these terms are problematic, because they use "White" as the criteria to lump all "nonWhite" racial groups into 1 category.[112] This is similar to defining working professional as veterinarians and nonveterinarians, which completely overlooks other fields.[112] The terms, *minority* and *colored*, have been used in the past but have lost popularity.[112] Author, historian, and antiracist, Ibram X. Kendi, expressed his thoughts about the term, *minority*. It made no sense as another name for Black people," he writes, "since most Black people lived, schooled, worked, socialized, and died in majority-Black spaces."[116,117] In a democracy, the majority decides while the minority dissents.[117] In the present society, the majority even gets to designate what kind of minority to be, that is, model minorities.[117]
   The most widely accepted and least problematic terms for racial groups are *POC*, *individuals of color*, and *communities of color*.[112] Another term are *Black, Indigenous*, and *POC* (BIPOC). As Richard Schaefer[118] summarized in his book, *Encyclopedia of Race, Ethnicity, and Society*, People of color, a political term, also is a term that allows for a more complex set of identity for the individual—a relational one that is in constant flux. However, when discussing an issue specific to a group, however, it is best to state the specific racial/ethnic community because it acknowledges and raises awareness of the group's history, that is, Nigerian American, Asian, and so forth.[112]
2. Hispanic/Latino/Latina/Latinx: *Latinx*, pronounced, "luh-TEE-neks," is a gender-neutral term used instead of Latino/Latina to refer to people in the United States whose cultural heritages can be traced to Central America and South America (collectively known as Latin America) or the Caribbean Islands.[112,119] This term refers to all people of Latin American descent and has become common in the LGBTQIA community because it is inclusive of all genders.[119] As Latinx grows in popularity, however, it also has become more controversial by the Latin American community for various reasons.

Table 2
Words and phrases that promote inclusion in the workplace[112]

Words to Avoid	Why They Should Be Avoided	More Inclusive Alternative Words
You guys	Associated with masculinity	You all, folks, friends, everyone, people
Handicap	This term may be rooted in a correlation between a disabled individual and a beggar.	Disabled
Ladies and gentlemen	Exclude those who are on the spectrum of gender and sexual orientation	Folks, my friends, people
Chairman, foreman	Associated with masculinity	Chairperson, chair, moderator, discussion leader
Housekeeping	This may feel gendered, specifically when referring to office work.	Maintenance, clean up
Husband, wife, boyfriend, girlfriend	Exclude those on the spectrum of gender and sexual orientation. May carry unwanted traditional implications of gender roles	Spouses, partners
Man hours, man the door, manpower	Associated with masculinity, suggests those who identify as men are productive and strong	Work, staff, or people/person
Cake walk, takes the cake	Slaves would perform dance in the nineteenth century to win a cake. Portrayed Black people as clumsily aspiring to be and dance like white people	That was easy
Crazy, nuts, insane, deranged, psycho, demented	These terms imply people with mental illnesses are "not normal."	Wild, surprising, unexpected
Lame	This is an ableism. Downplays the physical challenges of those who cannot walk	Uncool
Obsessive, compulsive, obsessive compulsive disorder	Using these mental health conditions to describe behavior undervalues the impact of the condition on those who live with it	Overly organized, particular
Mothering, fathering	Promote traditional gender roles, exclude nonbinary individuals	Parenting

(*continued on next page*)

Table 2 (continued)		
Words to Avoid	Why They Should Be Avoided	More Inclusive Alternative Words
Grandfathered in	The grandfather clause stated that back men could only vote if their parents or grandparents were able to vote before 1867.	Exempted from the new rule
Ghetto, barrio	Indicate a socially segregated urban nonwhite neighborhood	Rough, challenging. Or use the official name of the neighborhood you are describing

The term, *Hispanic*, has been used to refer to this diverse group of people and currently still is used by the US Census bureau; however, some individuals take issue with the term because it is appropriate to use when referring to people who are from Spain or have Spaniard ancestry.[112] Furthermore, misapplying the term can be offensive because it might imply a nod to Spanish colonialism.[112,119]

The terms, *Latino* and *Latina*, still commonly are used; however, the terms' gender connotations could be problematic for some members of the team.[112] Latinos typically is applied to the group as a whole and carries a masculine undertone.[112] Arguably, the preferred term is Latinx, especially among the millennial and Generation Z generations, which generally strive to be more gender-inclusive. Some individuals, however, may not mind being referred to as Latino or Latina.

3. *Native American/American Indian/Native/Indigenous American*: although these terms still cause some confusion, all these terms are acceptable.[112,120] American Indian or Indigenous American is preferred by many Native people, but the term American can be sensitive to some, because Native or Indigenous communities were established long before the land became known as America.[112] The term, Native American, however, is falling out of favor with some groups. When referring to Native or Indigenous people, it might be better to use their specific tribal names, such as Chickasaw, as long as the individual prefers this.[112]

4. Gender identity and sexual orientation: the use of gender-inclusive language means that language is used that does not discriminate against a particular sex or gender and does not perpetuate gender stereotypes.[121] As much as possible, nondiscriminatory language should be used, and each individual should be addressed using pronouns consistent with their gender identity.[121] More and more individuals are adding their preferred pronouns to public profiles and e-mail signatures in order to eliminate confusion and promote awareness around the tendency to misgender others.[112] In an effort to avoid marginalizing a teammate, they simply can be asked which gender they use.[112] Avoiding gender pronouns entirely or referring to teammates by their name also can be worked toward. He/him/his pronouns are used for individuals who identify as trangendered or cisgendered males and she/her/hers for transgendered or cisgendered females.[112] They/them/theirs refer to individuals who are nonbinary or gender fluid.[112]

Another helpful way to promote gender and sexual orientation inclusion is to avoid gender-biased expressions that reinforce gender stereotypes.[121] Men are URVM and often are inadvertently subjected to gender stereotypes, for instance, saying "men just don't understand" in a room of women and only 1 man.[121] Utilizing gender-neutral words also helps to enhance inclusiveness. For instance, "human-kind," "humanity," or "human race" is used instead of "mankind." Instead of addressing a group with "hello guys" or "hello ladies," modify with a simple, "Hello everyone."[121]

5. Learning to pronounce names: although diversity brings different types of talents, ideas, and identities to the team, it also brings different names. Names often carry cultural and family significance because names can connect children to their ancestors, country of origin, or ethnic group and often have deep significance for their families.[122] Learning to properly pronounce a teammate's names is an important part of showing them they are welcomed and valued. For many people with different names, mispronunciation of their name is one of the many ways their cultural heritage is disvalued.[122] The best way to learn to pronounce a name is to ask individuals directly and ask them how they say their names. They should not be asked what they wish to be called, because this indicates a preference for something "easier" to pronounce. The practice of racialized renaming has been going on since the seventeenth century, when Africans were forced to change their names and were given names of their masters.[122,123] And although forced renaming no longer is practiced, it is a common sentiment that nonWhite names are inconvenient and sometime unwelcome.[123] An effort should be made to ask for phonetic pronunciations of names and to permit the correction if unsure. If someone is unsure of how to pronounce another individual's name, it is not wrong to clarify how they would like to be addressed.

6. Ableism and Visible and Invisible Diversity: individuals with disability are a highly marginalized population.[124] In order to promote more acceptance, it commonly is encouraged to use people-first language when interacting with people from the disability community.[112] People-first language emphasizes the person, whose identity consists of a lot of things, one of which is a disability.[112] Using people-first language demonstrates a respect for the people with disabilities.[125] It demonstrates equality and recognition but also attempts to effect positive social change.[124] Using people-first language places the person before a phrase describing the person, for instance, "an individual with a disability" instead of a "disabled person" or "a child with autism" instead of an "autistic child."[124]

Identity-first language places the disability before the person. This is a controversial way of addressing individuals with disabilities. Some proponents of identity-first language state that individuals are demonstrating their acceptance and pride concerning their identities; thus, they are more likely to become a more autonomous individual.[124,126] As with any inclusive language, it usually is safest in following an individual's lead on how they choose to be addressed.[112]

Ableism is discrimination against individuals with a physical or mental disability. In order to avoid ableism, team members should avoid using terms like *blind*, *deaf*, *idiot*, *nuts*, or *psycho*.

Managing Holidays and Scheduling Conflicts

Team members need to be sensitive to other's cultural and religious obligations because individuals work together to achieve a common goal. Holidays are cultural events—some are religious and some are secular.[127] Although they differ in regard to the specifics of what and who is celebrated, religious and secular holidays revere particular individuals, events, and values.[127] Holidays serve as a cohesive function, binding people together through shared participation in rituals and celebrations.[127]

An example of a calendar of observances can be found at https://www.adl.org/education/resources/tools-and-strategies/calendar-of-observances.

The celebration of holidays in diverse society sometimes is problematic.[127] In some instances, government agencies give preference to holidays of some groups and not others.[127] An example is the difference in the way the Fourth of July and Emancipation Day or Thanksgiving and Kwanzaa are celebrated.[127] Another common problem is that 1 holiday may be a source of joy for some and a cause of sorrow for others, for instance, Pioneer Day as a celebration for Mormons but a day of sorrow for Native American Utes.[127] Indigenous Peoples' Day (Columbus Day) also is viewed differently by various groups.[127]

When decisions are made by the team about holidays (for instance who gets the day off and who gets to work), it is important to pay attention to the cultural or religious significance of the holiday to team members who have a strong opinion on what that holiday means to them.[127] When possible, team members should be flexible to allow others celebrate their cultural and religious obligations. Examples include individuals who cannot work on specific days or hours where they must observe Jewish holidays or the Sabbath.

When a majority of team members celebrate the same holidays, a rotating schedule could be created to ensure every individual gets an opportunity to get the day off. Religious or holiday preferences never should be used to discriminate against team members. This can be related to hiring practices or scheduling time off. For example, at 1 of the author's veterinary schools, Martin Luther King Day was the only holiday for which veterinary students had to make up missed classes. This created an unwelcoming environment for the 2 Black students enrolled in that veterinary school at that time.

Food in the Workplace

Food brings team members together and often is a great way to encourage and reward the team. With team diversity also comes the likelihood that there would be a wide variety of ethnic foods eaten at work by team members. The team should be sensitive to comments and reactions made around individuals eating different meals that might be culturally influenced. Instead of making comments about the smell of fragrant ethnic dishes in the break room, if bothered by the smell, team members may politely leave to eat somewhere else. Team members also should be sensitive to dietary restrictions of team members when planning events (ie, vegan and vegetarians) and also should be conscious of individuals who might need to fast at certain times.

Mentorship and Retaining Underrepresented Populations in Veterinary Medicine

Mentorship, an intense interpersonal relationship between a senior experienced colleague (mentor) and a less experienced colleague (protégé) is beneficial for all parties, including the mentor, protégé, and organization.[128] It has been shown that proteges typically have greater job successes, higher salaries, and enhanced career mobility. Mentors benefit from career enhancement, information exchange, and personal satisfaction, while organizations enjoy higher organization commitment and lower turnover.[128] Mentorship is critical to retaining diversity in the workplace. Studies have shown that women have less access to mentoring compared with men and POC report similar barriers to mentorship opportunities.[128–130]

Studies have shown that underrepresented individuals who advance the furthest share 1 characteristic: a strong network of mentors and cooperate sponsors.[131] Underrepresented individuals who achieved exceptional things at work enjoyed full developmental relationships with their mentors.[131] Individuals who are URVM should have access to mentorship and support from other individuals on the team. These mentors do not necessarily have to be URVM but mentors should have an understanding of the challenges faced by their mentees and should seek out ways to help their mentees overcome barriers to success in the organization. Education and guidance also should be available for these mentors (see previous section on diversity training) so that both individuals can develop an impactful relationship.

The small number of URVM, however, tends to compel them to serve as mentors to other URVM on the team. Too often, POC are expected to handle the affairs of other POC on the veterinary team and speak as the minority expert, while they get no support for their own roles on the team.[94] This may lead to little opportunity and support for the work that is valued by the organization (clinical service and research) and too much demand for work that is not rewarded (committee work or student club advisor).[93] Veterinary team leaders should ensure that their URVM employee is not overwhelmed by the task of participating in excessive amounts of activity structured around promoting diversity.

Communications with Diverse Individuals

Communications between individuals of varying demographics may range from simple to complex. The complexities may be deepened by differences in language, jargon, idioms, accents, and nonverbal cues. Having staff members who are multilingual is an incredible benefit, not only for diversifying the workplace but also for providing options to effectively communicate with clientele speaking the same language.[132] If a practice does not have the luxury of a bilingual staff member to act as a translator, Web-based language translators, such as Google Translate, can be used to assist in communications. Because pictures and visual media are universally understood, these tools may be employed in communications with diverse employees and clients. In addition, making the effort to learn another individual's language can be enlightening and respectful. Learning proper greetings or most commonly used phrases, such as "please" and "thank you," can be considered to create a more inclusive environment.

Team members should be sensitive to the cultural influences of communications, such as cultures that prohibit physical, verbal, or direct eye contact between individuals of opposite genders. People also should recognize that topics may be taboo to discuss with people of certain backgrounds.

Providing a Welcoming Space for all

In addition to changes that occur on an individual level, considerations for changes in the physical workspace also are helpful in celebrating diversity. Universal spaces, such as gender-neutral bathrooms and an interfaith space for meditation, reflection, and prayer, should be considered in an effort to make the workspace inviting to all. Offering only gendered bathrooms might make employees feel uncomfortable and might force them to make a choice that does not align with their gender identity. Having even 1 nongendered single-stall occupancy bathroom or creating universal multi-stall bathrooms provides an opportunity for transgendered individuals to feel accepted.[133] Having a quiet room where individuals of all cultural and religious background can relax, meditate, or pray also demonstrates to team members that the organization is committed to supporting every individual from all backgrounds.

Dealing with Conflicts with Respect and Acceptance

The authors realize that sometimes cultural views do not align, and members of the veterinary team may have strong feelings about certain issues that are against the strong feelings other team members have on the same issue.[134] For instance, different people and culture have different views on gender equality and gender roles.

When such conflicts arise, it often is a result of lack of understanding and respect for social or cultural differences. Creating opportunities for sincere open conversations about those issues may help raise awareness and increase understanding. Team members may have to agree to disagree on certain issues (as long as it does not create a hostile workplace for other team members), but the opposing viewpoints should be respected even when they cannot be accepted.

Implementing these recommendations at work in no doubt will celebrate the differences between team members and help everyone feel like they are part of the team. Team members should take personal action in self-education and growth. A list of questions that might help individuals and the team reflect on policies that promote inclusion in the workplace can be found at https://tanenbaum.org/programs/workplace/workplace-resources/religious-diversity-checklist/.

SUMMARY

Valuing diversity is critical in any workplace, and veterinary medicine is no exception.[135] Diversity is good for the veterinary clients and promotes a wholesome work environment for staff. There are numerous human attributes that contribute to diversity, and the inclusion of these varying attributes bring about numerous benefits in a working community. Continuous lifelong learning and further research on these topics are warranted to move the field forward to a more inclusive world.[1] Education and research in diversity and inclusion open the doors to alternative viewpoints and experiences and reduce stereotypes and discrimination. They encourage human beings to celebrate the similarities and embrace the differences between one another. Emphasizing these diversity issues will serve to boost an organization's reputation, expand clientele demographics, and improve employee satisfaction.

REFERENCES

1. Roberson QM. Diversity in the workplace: a review, synthesis, and future research agenda. Annual review of organizational psychology and organizational behavior. 2019;6:69–88.

2. Stevens FG, Plaut VC, Sanchez-Burks J. Unlocking the benefits of diversity: all-inclusive multiculturalism and positive organizational change. J Appl Behav Sci 2008;44(1):116–33.

3. Brief AP. Diversity at work. Cambridge (United Kingdom): Cambridge University Press; 2008.

4. Earley CP, Mosakowski E. Creating hybrid team cultures: an empirical test of transnational team functioning. Acad Manage J 2000;43(1):26–49.

5. M S. Is self-leadership the best leadership? Ritz-Carlton's emplyee emplowerment. Available at: https://www.forbes.com/sites/micahsolomon/2014/05/13/ritz-carltons-corporate-culture/?sh=182e95c6f6e6. Accessed January 11, 2021.

6. Ruby K, Stone D. What makes a veterinary team. Clinician's Brief 2013;4.

7. Peduzzi M. Multiprofessional healthcare team: concept and typology. Rev Saude Publica 2001;35:103–9.

8. Katzenbach JR, Smith DK. The wisdom of teams: creating the high-performance organization. Brighton (MA): Harvard Business Review Press; 2015.

9. Moore IC, Coe JB, Adams CL, et al. The role of veterinary team effectiveness in job satisfaction and burnout in companion animal veterinary clinics. J Am Vet Med Assoc 2014;245(5):513–24.

10. Borrill CS, Carletta J, Carter A, et al. The effectiveness of health care teams in the National Health Service. University of Aston in Birmingham Birmingham; 2000.

11. Mickan S, Rodger S. Characteristics of effective teams: a literature review. Aust Health Rev 2000;23(3):201–8.

12. Mickan SM, Rodger SA. Effective health care teams: a model of six characteristics developed from shared perceptions. J Interprof Care 2005;19(4):358–70.

13. Lemieux-Charles L, McGuire WL. What do we know about health care team effectiveness? A review of the literature. Med Care Res Rev 2006;63(3): 263–300.

14. Cyr A. Diversity dominates Carabins soccer team. Available at: https://usports. ca/en/sports/soccer/m/news/2017/10/2096994016/diversity-dominates-carabins-soccer-teams. Accessed January 11, 2021.

15. Wambui TW, Wangombe JG, Muthura MW, et al. Managing workplace diversity: a Kenyan perspective. Int J Bus Soc Sci 2013;4(16):199–218.

16. George Washington University. Office for Diversity EaCE. Diveristy and inclusion defined. Available at: https://diversity.gwu.edu/diversity-and-inclusion-defined. Accessed January 11, 2021.

17. AAVMC. Definition of Diversity. Available at: https://www.aavmc.org/assets/Site_ 18/files/About_AAVMC/Definition%20of%20Diversity%20(ID%2099548).pdf. Accessed January 13, 2020.

18. Annie E Casey Foundation. Equity vs. equality and other racial justice definitions. Available at: https://www.aecf.org/blog/racial-justice-definitions/? gclid=Cj0KCQiA0fr_BRDaARIsAABw4EtMr8nHwHzeIGnA3pEAiyRsAchTdRq BheZX3jlHTmFrzzHA6pK75xkaAoDEEALw_wcB. Accessed January 13, 2021.

19. United States Census Bureau. Population by Race in the United States. Available at: https://data.census.gov/cedsci/profile?q=United%20States&g= 0100000US. Accessed January 13, 2021.

20. Strmic-Pawl HV, Jackson BA, Garner S. Race counts: racial and ethnic data on the US census and the implications for tracking inequality. Sociol Race Ethn 2018;4(1):1–13.

21. Tusty M, Flores B, Victor R, et al. The long "race" to diversity in otolaryngology. Otolaryngol Head Neck Surg 2021;164(1):6–8.

22. Gonsiorek JC, Sell RL, Weinrich JD. Definition and measurement of sexual orientation. Suicide Life Threat Behav 1995;25:40–51.

23. Nagoshi JL, Brzuzy SI, Terrell HK. Deconstructing the complex perceptions of gender roles, gender identity, and sexual orientation among transgender individuals. Feminism & Psychology 2012;22(4):405–22.

24. Wilchins R, Nestle J, Howell C, et al. GenderQueer-voices from beyond the sexual binary. Riverdale (NY): Riverdale Avenue Books LLC; 2020.

25. Bailey JM, Vasey PL, Diamond LM, et al. Sexual orientation, controversy, and science. Psychol Sci Publ Interest 2016;17(2):45–101.

26. Glossary of terms related to sexuality and gender. 2003. Available at: http:// www.columbia.org/pdf_files/glossary_of_sexuality_and_gender.pdf. Accessed January 13, 2021.

27. Center for Educational Justice and Community Engagement University of California B. Definition of Terms. Available at: https://cejce.berkeley.edu/ geneq/resources/lgbtq-resources/definition-terms. Accessed January 13, 2021.

28. Americans with Disability Act (ADA). A guide to disability rights laws. Available at: https://www.ada.gov/cguide.htm#anchor62335. Accessed January 11, 2021.

29. World Health Organization. World report on disability. 2011. Available at: https://www.who.int/teams/noncommunicable-diseases/disability-and-rehabilitation/world-report-on-disability. Accessed January 11, 2021.

30. Boehm SA, Dwertmann DJ. Forging a single-edged sword: facilitating positive age and disability diversity effects in the workplace through leadership, positive climates, and HR practices. Work, Aging and Retirement 2015;1(1):41–63.

31. Von Schrader S, Malzer V, Bruyère S. Perspectives on disability disclosure: the importance of employer practices and workplace climate. Employee Responsibilities and Rights Journal 2014;26(4):237–55.

32. Phillips BN, Deiches J, Morrison B, et al. Disability diversity training in the workplace: systematic review and future directions. J Occup Rehabil 2016;26(3):264–75.

33. Muyia Nafukho F, Roessler RT, Kacirek K. Disability as a diversity factor: implications for human resource practices. Adv Dev Hum Resour 2010;12(4):395–406.

34. Steil JM, Makowski DG. Equity, equality, and need: a study of the patterns and outcomes associated with their use in intimate relationships. Soc Justice Res 1989;3(2):121–37.

35. Grigg EK, Hart LA. Enhancing success of veterinary visits for clients with disabilities and an assistance dog or companion animal: a review. Front Vet Sci 2019;6:44.

36. Morin EC. Americans with disabilities act of 1990: social integration through employment. Cath UL Rev 1990;40:189.

37. AAVMC guidelines for service animal access to veterinary teaching facilities. 2019. Available at: https://www.aavmc.org/assets/Site_18/files/About_AAVMC/Service_Animal_Access.pdf. Accessed January 11, 2021.

38. American Psychological Association TFoSS. Report of the APA task force on socioeconomic status. Washington, DC: Author; 2007.

39. Williams DR, Mohammed SA, Leavell J, et al. Race, socioeconomic status and health: complexities, ongoing challenges and research opportunities. Ann N Y Acad Sci 2010;1186:69.

40. Wyatt-Nichol H, Brown S, Haynes W. Social class and socioeconomic status: relevance and inclusion in MPA-MPP programs. J Public Aff 2011;17(2):187–208.

41. Ellison SF, Mullin WP. Diversity, social goods provision, and performance in the firm. J Econ Manag Strat 2014;23(2):465–81.

42. Park JJ, Denson N, Bowman NA. Does socioeconomic diversity make a difference? Examining the effects of racial and socioeconomic diversity on the campus climate for diversity. Am Educ Res J 2013;50(3):466–96.

43. Martin SR, Côté S. Social class transitioners: their cultural abilities and organizational importance. Springfield (MA): Acad Manage Rev 2019;44(3):618–42.

44. Webster M. Dictionary and thesaurus. (CD-ROM) Merriam Webster; 2014.

45. Purdue University Global. Generational differences in the workplace [Infographic]. Available at: https://www.purdueglobal.edu/education-partnerships/generational-workforce-differences-infographic/. Accessed January 11, 2021.

46. Boehm SA, Kunze F. Age diversity and age climate in the workplace. Aging workers and the employee-employer relationship. Springer; 2015. p. 33–55.

47. Riach K. Managing 'difference': understanding age diversity in practice. Human Resource Management Journal 2009;19(3):319–35.

48. U.S. Department of Labor. Age discrimination. Available at: https://www.dol.gov/general/topic/discrimination/agedisc#:~:text=The%20Age%20Discrimination%20in%20Employment,conditions%20or%20privileges%20of%20employment. Accessed January 11, 2021.

49. Ilmakunnas P, Ilmakunnas S. Diversity at the workplace: whom does it benefit? Economist 2011;159(2):223–55.

50. Burmeister A, Wang M, Hirschi A. Understanding the motivational benefits of knowledge transfer for older and younger workers in age-diverse coworker dyads: an actor–partner interdependence model. J Appl Psychol 2020;105(7): 748–59.

51. Wang M, Fang Y. Age diversity in the workplace: facilitating opportunities with organizational practices. Public Policy & Aging Report 2020;30(3):119–23.

52. Laperrière M, Lépinard E. Intersectionality as a tool for social movements: strategies of inclusion and representation in the Québécois women's movement. Politics 2016;36(4):374–82.

53. Hunting G, Grace D, Hankivsky O. Taking action on stigma and discrimination: an intersectionality-informed model of social inclusion and exclusion. Intersectionalities: A Global Journal of Social Work Analysis, Research, Polity, and Practice. 2015;4(2):101–25.

54. Cho S, Crenshaw KW, McCall L. Toward a field of intersectionality studies: theory, applications, and praxis. Signs (Chic) 2013;38(4):785–810.

55. Crenshaw K. Demarginalizing the intersection of race and sex: a Black feminist critique of antidiscrimination doctrine, feminist theory and antiracist politics. New York: u Chi Legal f; 1989. p. 139.

56. YW Boston Blog. What is intersectionality, and what does it have to do with me?. Available at: https://www.ywboston.org/2017/03/what-is-intersectionality-and-what-does-it-have-to-do-with-me/. Accessed January 11, 2021.

57. Brand S. Whole earth discipline. London (UK): Atlantic Books Ltd; 2010.

58. Douglas PS, Williams KA, Walsh MN. Diversity matters. Washington, DC: American College of Cardiology Foundation; 2017.

59. Williamson IO, Slay HS, Shapiro DL, et al. The effect of explanations on prospective applicants reactions to firm diversity practices. Human Resource Management: Published in Cooperation with the School of Business Administration, The University of Michigan and in alliance with the Society of Human Resources Management. 2008;47(2):311–30.

60. Moore FA, Johnson M, Perry W, et al. Why racial and ethnic diversity in residency matters. Emerg Med News 2016;38(7):3–4.

61. Komaromy M, Grumbach K, Drake M, et al. The role of Black and Hispanic physicians in providing health care for underserved populations. N Engl J Med 1996;334(20):1305–10.

62. Kahler SC. The changing face of the profession. J Am Vet Med Assoc 2010;236: 368–9.

63. Kornegay LM. A business case for diversity and inclusion: why it is important for veterinarians to embrace our changing communities. J Am Vet Med Assoc 2011; 238(9):1103–5.

64. Bernstein R, Edwards T. An older and more diverse nation by midcentury. US Census Bureau News 2008;14.

65. Cross T. Veterinary medicine: the most racially segregated field in graduate education today. The Journal of Blacks in Higher Education 2003;42:8–19.

66. Dabdub DL. Diversity and inclusion in veterinary medicine. Advisor 2020; 40(3):1–3.

67. Elmore RG. The lack of racial diversity in veterinary medicine. J Am Vet Med Assoc 2003;222(1):24–6.
68. LaVallee E, Mueller MK, McCobb E. A systematic review of the literature addressing veterinary care for underserved communities. J Appl Anim Welf Sci 2017;20(4):381–94.
69. Greenhill LM, Nelson PD, Elmore RG. Racial, cultural, and ethnic diversity within US veterinary colleges. J Vet Med Educ 2007;34(2):74–8.
70. Association of American Veterinary Medical Colleges. Annual data report 2019-2020 (Internet). 2020:1-64. Available at: http://www.aavmc.org/About-AAVMC/Public-Data.aspx. Accessed January 11, 2021.
71. Chadderdon LM, Lloyd JW, Pazak HE. New directions for veterinary technology. J Vet Med Educ 2014;41(1):96–101.
72. Norkus CL, Liss DJ, Leighton LS. Characteristics of the labor market for veterinary technician specialists in 2013. J Am Vet Med Assoc 2016;248(1):105–9.
73. Rivers FGB. # BlackLivesMatter to all of us. Vet Rec 2020;186(18):613.
74. Evans MK, Rosenbaum L, Malina D, et al. Diagnosing and treating systemic racism. N Engl J Med 2020;383(3):274–6.
75. Sexton SM, Richardson CR, Schrager SB, et al. Systemic racism and health disparities: a statement from editors of family medicine journals. Ann Fam Med 2021;19(1):2.
76. McCluney CL, King DD, Bryant CM, et al. From "calling in Black" to "calling for antiracism resources": the need for systemic resources to address systemic racism. Equality, Diversity and Inclusion: An International Journal 2020;40(1):49–59.
77. Walker GT Jr, Taylor MA, Chansky HA. What's important: take a knee: our collective responsibility to dismantle systemic racism. J Bone Joint Surg Am 2020;103(1):92–4.
78. Multicultural Veterinary Medical Association. Wake up, Vet Med. 2020. Available at: https://www.mcvma.org/wakeup. Accessed January 11, 2021.
79. Irvine L, Vermilya JR. Gender work in a feminized profession: the case of veterinary medicine. Gend Soc 2010;24(1):56–82.
80. Jones SD. Valuing animals: veterinarians and their patients in modern America. Baltimore (MD): JHU Press; 2003.
81. Larsen PH. Our history of women in veterinary medicine: gumption. grace, grit and good humor. Littleton (CO): Association for Women Veterinarians; 1997.
82. American Veterinary Medical Association. Schaumburg (IL): AVMA report on compensation; 2007.
83. Waite S. Should I stay or should I go? Employment discrimination and workplace harassment against transgender and other minority Employees in Canada's Federal Public Service. J Homosex 2020;1–27.
84. Romanelli M, Lindsey MA. Patterns of healthcare discrimination among transgender help-seekers. Am J Prev Med 2020;58(4):e123–31.
85. Boustani K, Taylor KA. Navigating LGBTQ+ discrimination in academia: where do we go from here? Biochemist 2020;42(3):16–20.
86. Ullman J. Present, yet not welcomed: gender diverse teachers' experiences of discrimination. Teach Education 2020;31(1):67–83.
87. Griner SB, Vamos CA, Thompson EL, et al. The intersection of gender identity and violence: victimization experienced by transgender college students. J Interpers Violence 2020;35(23–24):5704–25.

88. Cogan C M, Scholl JA, Lee JY, et al. Sexual violence and suicide risk in the transgender population: the mediating role of proximal stressors. Psychol Sex 2020;12(1):1–12.

89. Yi S, Chann N, Chhoun P, et al. Social marginalization, gender-based violence, and binge drinking among transgender women in Cambodia. Drug Alcohol Depend 2020;207:107802.

90. Mak J, Shires DA, Zhang Q, et al. Suicide attempts among a cohort of transgender and gender diverse people. Am J Prev Med 2020;59(4):570–7.

91. Budge SL. Suicide and the transgender experience: a public health crisis. Am Psychol 2020;75(3):380.

92. Cerel J, Tucker RR, Aboussouan A, et al. Suicide exposure in transgender and gender diverse adults. J Affect Disord 2020;278:165–71.

93. Turner CSV. Women of color in academe: living with multiple marginality. The Journal of Higher Education 2002;73(1):74–93.

94. Laden BV, Hagedorn LS. Job satisfaction among faculty of color in academe: individual survivors or institutional transformers? New Directions for Institutional Research 2000;2000(105):57–66.

95. Center for Excellence for Diversity and Inclusion in Veterinary Medicine. Certificates for Diverstiy and Inclusion in Veterinary Medicine. Purdue Universtiy College of Veterinary Medicine. Available at: https://vet.purdue.edu/humancenteredvetmed/overview.php. Accessed February 14, 2021.

96. Center for Creative Leadership. 5 Powerful Ways to Take REAL Action on DEI (Diversity, Equity & Inclusion). Available at: https://www.ccl.org/articles/leading-effectively-articles/5-powerful-ways-to-take-real-action-on-dei-diversity-equity-inclusion/. Accessed February 14, 2021.

97. Bonilla-Silva E. The structure of racism in color-blind, "post-racial" America. Los Angeles (CA): Sage Publications Sage CA; 2015.

98. Day JC, Newburger EC. The big payoff: educational attainment and synthetic estimates of work-life earnings. special studies. Washington, DC: Current Population Reports; 2002.

99. Pager D. The use of field experiments for studies of employment discrimination: contributions, critiques, and directions for the future. Ann Am Acad Pol Soc Sci 2007;609(1):104–33.

100. Pager D, Quillian L. Walking the talk? What employers say versus what they do. Am Sociol Rev 2005;70(3):355–80.

101. Castilla EJ, Benard S. The paradox of meritocracy in organizations. Adm Sci Q 2010;55(4):543–676.

102. Sendaula S. Black fatigue: how racism erodes the mind, body, and spirit. New York: Reed Business Information; 2020. 360 Park Avenue South.

103. Ray V. A theory of racialized organizations. Am Sociol Rev 2019;84(1):26–53.

104. Castilla EJ. Achieving meritocracy in the workplace. MIT Sloan Management Review 2016;57(4):35.

105. Togoh Isabel. Michael Seibel Becomes Reddit's First Black Board Member After Alexis Ohanian's Resignation. Forbes. 2020. Available at: https://www.forbes.com/sites/isabeltogoh/2020/06/10/michael-seibel-becomes-reddits-first-black-board-member-after-alexis-ohanians-resignation/?sh=25b4f632430a. Accessed January 11, 2021.

106. Aveling N. Anti-racism in schools: A question of leadership? Discourse: studies in the cultural politics of education. 2007;28(1):69–85.

107. Blanchard FA, Crandall CS, Brigham JC, et al. Condemning and condoning racism: a social context approach to interracial settings. J Appl Psychol 1994; 79(6):993.

108. X KI. This is what an antiracist America would look like. How do we get there? The Guardian. 2018. Available at: https://www.theguardian.com/commentisfree/2018/dec/06/antiracism-and-america-white-nationalism.

109. Kendi IX. How to be an antiracist. London (UK): One World; 2019. Accessed January 11, 2021.

110. Mandel H, Semyonov M. Going back in time? Gender differences in trends and sources of the racial pay gap, 1970 to 2010. Am Sociol Rev 2016;81(5): 1039–68.

111. Weinberg M. LGBT-inclusive language. English Journal 2009;98(4):50.

112. Mulki S, Stone-Sabali S. Using inclusive language in the workplace. Journal AWWA 2020;112(11):64–70.

113. Lauring J, Klitmøller A. Inclusive language use in multicultural business organizations: the effect on creativity and performance. International Journal of Business Communication 2017;54(3):306–24.

114. Bourke J. The diversity and inclusion revolution: eight powerful truths. 2018. Available at: https://www2.deloitte.com/us/en/insights/deloitte-review/issue-22/diversity-and-inclusion-at-work-eight-powerful-truths.html/#endnote-18. Accessed January 11, 2021.

115. Linguistic Society of America. Available at: https://www.linguisticsociety.org/. Accessed January 11, 2021.

116. Kendi IX. Stamped from the beginning: the definitive history of racist ideas in America. Random House; 2017.

117. Morris W. Is Being a 'Minority' Really Just a Matter of Numbers? New York Times Magazine. Available at: https://www.nytimes.com/2019/01/23/magazine/is-being-a-minority-really-just-a-matter-of-numbers.html. Accessed January 11, 2021.

118. Schaefer RT, Thousand Oaks CA. Encyclopedia of race, ethnicity, and society, vol. 1. Sage; 2008.

119. Rodriguez A. 'Latinx' explained: a history of the controversial word and how to pronounce it. USA Today. Available at: https://www.usatoday.com/story/news/nation/2019/06/29/latina-latino-latinx-hispanic-what-do-they-mean/1596501001/. Accessed January 11, 2021.

120. Horse PG. Native American identity. New Dir Student Serv 2005; 2005(109):61–8.

121. Guidelines for gender-inclusive language in English. Available at: https://www.un.org/en/gender-inclusive-language/guidelines.shtml. Accessed January 11, 2021.

122. Kohli R, Solórzano DG. Teachers, please learn our names!: racial microaggressions and the K-12 classroom. Race Ethn Educ 2012;15(4):441–62.

123. Dillard J. Black names.-the Hague, vol. 118. Mouton & Co., Publishers; 1976. p. 1976.

124. Flink P. Person-first & identity-first language: supporting students with disabilities on campus. Community Coll J Res Pract 2021;45(2):79–85.

125. Clarke LS, Embury DC, Knight C, et al. People-first language, equity, and inclusion: how do we say it, and why does it matter? Learning disabilities: a multidisciplinary journal. 2017;22(1):74–9.

126. Dunn DS, Andrews EE. Person-first and identity-first language: developing psychologists' cultural competence using disability language. Am Psychol 2015; 70(3):255.

127. Naylor DT, Smith BD. Holidays, cultural diversity, and the public culture. Washington, DC: ERIC; 1997. p. 257.

128. Smith JW, Smith WJ, Markham SE. Diversity issues in mentoring academic faculty. J Career Dev 2000;26(4):251–62.

129. Kram KE. Mentoring at work: developmental relationships in organizational life. Washington, DC: University Press of America; 1988.

130. Thomas DA. Racial dynamics in cross-race developmental relationships. Adm Sci Q 1993;169–94.

131. Thomas DA. The truth about mentoring minorities. Race matters. Harv Bus Rev 2001;79(4):98–107, 168.

132. Tange H, Lauring J. Language management and social interaction within the multilingual workplace. J Comm Manag 2009;13(3):218–31.

133. Designing for Inclusivity. Strategies for Universal Washrooms and Change Rooms. 2018. Available at: http://hcma.ca/wp-content/uploads/2018/01/HCMA_Designing-for-Inclusivity_V1-1.pdf.

134. Yadav R. Cross-cultural conflicts. 2018. Accessed January 11, 2021.

135. Kiefer V, Grogan KB, Chatfield J, et al. Cultural competence in veterinary practice. J Am Vet Med Assoc 2013;243(3):326–8.

Compassion Fatigue
Understanding Empathy

Kelly Harrison, DVM, MS

KEYWORDS

- Empathy • Compassion fatigue • Veterinary medicine

KEY POINTS

- Empathy is central to good medical practice; empathetic display affects client, patient, and provider well-being; empathy and compassion fatigue are intertwined and can be associated with negative mental health outcome for veterinarians.

INTRODUCTION

The subject of empathy in the context of clinical practice is an area of increasing research interest. The concept of empathy has been described as one that is intuitively understood, until you try to define it.[1] Empathy is thought to be a central aspect of caretaking and may be considered one of the most important characteristics exhibited by health care providers in terms of patient perception, as well as positive health outcomes.[2-5] Empathy has been defined as an educational objective in medical training programs worldwide, as increased awareness of patient perception and the development of a holistic and patient-centered approach is being prioritized.[6-10] According to the Institute of Medicine, empathy also plays an important role in achieving patient-centeredness, as 1 of the 6 main goals of a twenty-first century health care system, which comprises the "*qualities of compassion, empathy, and responsiveness to the needs, values, and expressed preferences of the individual patient*".[11] Generally regarded as the capacity to understand and share feelings of another, empathy allows us to vicariously feel the joy, or alternatively pain, associated with an experience.[12] Importantly, when experiencing empathy one feels *with* someone but does not equate one's own feelings with another's.[12]

BACKGROUND

Whether or not characteristics of empathy are innate, learned, or a combination of both remains unclear. It has been proposed that an empathetic response is produced by 1 or both of 2 functional systems; one system is automatic, develops early, and is

University of Florida College of Veterinary Medicine, 2015 Southwest 16thAvenue, Gainesville, FL 32608, USA
E-mail address: kelmeyer@ufl.edu

Vet Clin Small Anim 51 (2021) 1041–1051
https://doi.org/10.1016/j.cvsm.2021.04.020
vetsmall.theclinics.com
0195-5616/21/© 2021 Elsevier Inc. All rights reserved.

seen in a variety of species, whereas the other involves controlled processing, develops later, and may be a unique feature of the human species.[13] Empathy is not typically thought of as reflex, although it might begin as one, rather it is a way of understanding.[14] It has been suggested that the idea of empathy depends on context as well as an individual's *motives* in relation to context.[15] In addition, findings suggest that people want to empathize with those most relevant to them.[15] *Empathetic motives* are internal forces that drive an individual's desire to engage or separate from social connection and are often linked to specific goals.[15] Brain studies of empathy have attributed different social responses to more than 10 different areas of the cortex and limbic system known as the "empathy circuit" of the human brain.[16,17]

EMPATHY IN HEALTH CARE

In clinical medicine, empathy has been defined as *the ability to understand the patient's situation, perspective, and feelings and to communicate that understanding back to the patient.*[18] Empathy is also a feeling of being *seen.*[19] In veterinary medicine, these principles are applicable to the clients we serve and the patients we care for. A source of confusion can be found when *empathy* is used interchangeably or overlaps in definition with the terms *sympathy* and *compassion.*[20] In general, sympathy is defined as an emotional reaction of feeling pity toward the misfortune of another, whereas compassion recognizes these hardships and then takes actions to help.[21,22] Alternatively, empathy is defined as the ability to understand and acknowledge the feelings of another.[23,24] How a client or patient defines and perceives the terms *empathy*, *sympathy*, and *compassion* in a clinical setting is not well known. Often, a patient who perceives empathy by a health care provider will be satisfied with their care regardless of whether or not something can be done, or alternatively, when a mistake is made.[14] This, in itself, highlights the importance of communication in a clinical setting and how the perception of care can either be promoted or be precluded by feelings of empathy. On the human side palliative care patients were able to distinguish characteristics between the terms *empathy*, *sympathy*, and *compassion*, offering preferences relative to one another, specifically a preference for compassion and empathy over sympathy.[20]

DISPLAY OF EMPATHY

Expression of empathy requires some degree of social skill and can be expressed both verbally and nonverbally. Posture, eye contact, facial expressions, and body movements are all examples of nonverbal empathy.[25,26] In particular, direction of gaze and body orientation have been shown to have positive and/or negative effect on the perception of empathy.[27] Awareness of culture-based norms such as race, nationality, sex, and gender also affect expectations of nonverbal expressions as they pertain to the perception of empathy.[28] Communication of empathy may be verbal or nonverbal in origin, and although recognized as important, its total impact is difficult to measure.[29–33] In a clinical setting, empathy has been further characterized by 4 different components:

1. Affective: the ability to experience patient or client emotions
2. Moral: the internal incentive to empathize
3. Cognitive: the intellectual ability to identify and comprehend others' perspectives and emotions
4. Behavioral: the ability to understand and convey these emotions and perspectives back to the patient or the client[34]

Acquiring a better understanding of these different dimensions may help to define specific elements that contribute to positive and negative indicators of empathy.

ASSESSMENT OF EMPATHY

Assessment of empathy in a clinical setting is difficult. Multiple systems for assessing empathy have been described, and yet the majority have little power to predict the presence or absence of empathy in a clinical setting.[35] The most commonly used measurement for assessing empathy was self-reporting, yet multiple studies have found that self-reports of empathetic display are only loosely correlated with behavior and patient perception.[35–39] Lack of a universal definition, a mismatch between definition and defined measurements, and an overreliance on cognition and self-reporting are limitations associated with evaluating empathy in a medical setting.[35] A patient's perception of their relationship with health care professionals greatly affects the degree of reported empathy, which has inspired new tools for evaluating empathy in a clinical setting, taking into consideration patient perspective.[40,41] Although more research is required to validate assessments of empathy in a medical setting, it is reasonable to consider that any measurement or description of clinical empathy should include terms of patient perception.

For studies that measure empathy, high scores have been associated with professionalism, clinical competency, confidence, and well-being.[42–44] In human and veterinary medicine, a patient or client's perception of empathy can influence clinical outcomes including greater patient satisfaction, regulation of patient symptoms, as well as compliance with medical recommendations.[45–54] Empathy displayed by physicians has also been shown to promote the sharing and disclosure of significant information by patients.[51,52]

THE COST OF EMPATHY

Although the demonstration of empathy has the potential to have a positive impact to the patient, it also has the potential to affect the provider. For health care providers these interactions may leave a positive or negative impression. In a clinical setting, empathy is often demonstrated in situations of pain and suffering. These expressions of an empathetic response to suffering have the potential to result in 2 separate outcomes: empathetic concern (compassion) or empathetic distress (personal distress).[12] Empathetic concern (compassion) is a natural response to elicit helping behavior when observing another's distress.[55] In response to suffering and as a way to prevent excessive sharing, one may respond with compassion instead of empathy.[12] Compassion initiates action and embodies feelings of warmth, care, and concern and is characterized by feeling *for* someone rather than feeling *with* someone.[12] Compassion is associated with feelings of love and results in good health and prosocial motivation. Empathetic distress refers to a strongly aversive and self-oriented response to the suffering of others, accompanied by a desire to withdraw oneself from a situation with the goal of protection from it.[12] Feelings of empathetic distress may negatively affect a clinician's well-being, as they attempt to internalize the emotional pain and distress of others. These feelings can build, leading to poor health and emotional and social withdrawal.

The term *compassion fatigue* has been used to describe different forms of emotional, physical, or behavioral distress associated with acts of caring; however, a precise definition remains inconsistent. Compassion fatigue is a broadly defined concept that is typically associated with caregiving in which people or animals are experiencing significant emotional or physical pain and suffering.[56] It has been described in a variety of disciplines, and its definition can often be found overlapping with other commonly associated terms such as burnout, ethical fatigue, moral distress, and secondary traumatic stress. Compassion fatigue has been described as a set of symptoms, rather than a disease, and can manifest as emotional, behavioral, and/or physical distress. Symptoms of compassion fatigue may include, but are not limited to, dissociation, numbness, isolation, hypervigilance, sleep problems, tearfulness, avoidance, and/or obsession and often develop over time.[57] Chronic expression of empathy and compassion fatigue are intertwined, but a clear delineation of their impact on the mental health and well-being of veterinary professionals is not well understood. Highlighting what is known about this relationship may serve as a foundation to better combat the undesirable, and often harmful, effects veterinarians may endure in their role as caretakers.

It has been proposed that exhibiting clinical empathy may, in itself, over time contribute to compassion fatigue and emotional exhaustion.[58–60] As a result, some physicians have actually aimed for a version of empathy that strives to understand the needs of the patient while "detaching" emotionally in order to make difficult decisions in an unobstructed manner but also as a form of protection to mitigate the risk of compassion fatigue and burnout.[19] Duarte and Pinto-Gouveia connected the concept of empathy-derived guilt in nurses as a detriment to professional quality of life and found that those with more empathetic feelings of care and concern may be more vulnerable to experience burnout and symptoms of compassion fatigue.[59] Empathy-based guilt becomes pathologic when it leads to cognitive errors in understanding causality; in other words, when people who feel empathy falsely believe they have either caused or have the means to relieve the person of suffering but have failed to do so.[59] It has been suggested that empathic concern may have a point in which a positive experience of caring for another may transition into having a personal and traumatic effect.[61] It is reasonable to assume that continued and repetitive exposure to experiences that evoke empathy may negatively affect professional satisfaction and emotional well-being. In some ways, this concept can be looked on as the idea of *compassion resilience*, where knowledge and awareness are the key components to managing these situations. Understanding the dynamic relationship between empathetic display and how it affects caretaker's quality of life may provide valuable strategies to mitigate negative outcomes for health care professionals. In addition, it may also help to improve the sustainability of medical professionals whose jobs require some degree of emotional investment as part of a comprehensive approach to medicine.

EMPATHY AND PROFESSIONAL STUDENTS

Interestingly, there are identifiable trends when it comes to empathy in professional students. A systematic review of 18 studies investigating empathy during medical school and some residency programs found that self-perceived empathy decreases significantly over the course of these training programs.[52] These findings are consistent with previously published evidence-based longitudinal studies.[62–69] In particular, an association between a decline in empathy and an increase in patient contact during the clinical phases of training was observed. These findings may demonstrate that increasing demands for displays of empathy can negatively affect the provider by causing a subsequent decrease in their ability to express empathy. It is reasonable to assume that factors such as mental exhaustion, lack of productive coping skills, and limitations in resiliency also play a role. In a similar study, personal distress, defined as self-oriented feelings of anxiety and unease, was measured in veterinary students and found to gradually increase as they progressed through the curriculum and assumed greater responsibility for client communication and patient care.[34] One concerning finding is that these feelings may carry over from an academic setting to a professional setting. In 2004, a study of veterinary interactions reported that practicing veterinarians expressed empathy in only 7% of appointments.[70] Additional factors that may contribute to a decrease in empathy and increase in personal distress in a clinical setting may include interpersonal challenges with superiors or mentors, increased responsibilities and workload, increased client/patient communication, and a shift from the idealism and enthusiasm of medicine to objectivity and technology.[63–65,71–73] Because of the extreme time commitments and levels of stress often experienced in a clinical setting, it can be assumed that the loss or disruption of the passion for one's profession is detrimental to their overall well-being. Similarly, having little in the way of resources to effectively identify and manage symptoms of compassion fatigue and burnout may further contribute to ones' professional dissatisfaction. Increasing awareness of the interactions that contribute to these sequelae and creating a plan is critical to long-term success and happiness; incorporating training opportunities early within the confines of the professional curricula may improve long-term outcomes.

EMPATHY AND EMOTIONAL INTELLIGENCE

The ability to recognize the emotions of oneself and another, using emotions to guide thought and behavior, and an understanding of how emotions shape behavior and emotional regulation is known as *emotional intelligence*.[74] Empathy is considered an interpersonal skill and is one of the many components of assessing ones' score in emotional intelligence.[75] A 2020 study of fourth year veterinary students and house officers found that emotional intelligence scores were predominately less than the mean of other professionals at all stages of training and did not increase over time.[75] Other studies point to an overall decline in empathy as well as few opportunities to learn how to practice empathy within the veterinary curriculum.[34,76] Furthermore, another study found that personal distress scores, a negative indicator of empathy, seem to increase throughout veterinary school and are highest in new graduates compared with colleagues with 20 years or more of experience.[34] A lack of social support and increasing isolation while transitioning from veterinary school to clinical practice is thought to contribute to these outcomes.[77] These findings suggest an effort to maintain or improve emotional skillsets may be warranted as part of a veterinary curriculum and could contribute to improvements in work place stressors as well as professional satisfaction following graduation.

PERSONAL DISTRESS

Personal distress, thought to be a measure of affective empathy, has been associated with increased frequency of self-perceived medical errors.[67] When experienced chronically, this type of distress may contribute to negative health outcomes for patients,[12] and this may be the result of a decrease in patient sharing and compliance or alternatively the fact that personal distress, itself, has been linked with increased odds of future medical errors.[34] It is reasonable to assume that an increase in personal distress negatively affects the well-being of health care professionals. In the veterinary profession, numerous studies have linked veterinarians with anxiety, depression, and suicidal ideation.[78–83] Depression and personal distress observed in medical students improved over the course of residency training; however, an initial decline in empathy remained low throughout the course of the residency.[66] It has been suggested that shielding oneself from identifying with another's distress, expressed as a decline in empathy, may be a coping mechanism for dealing with excessive emotional stimulation.[58] A lack of clinical empathy in physicians has been associated with burnout and emotional exhaustion, but the exact causality remains unclear.[58] A better understanding of the components that shape empathy in doctor-patient interactions may give health care professionals an advantage in mitigating personal struggles with mental health. Furthermore, deconstructing the relationships between compassion fatigue, empathy, and caretaking in a clinical setting may positively affect patient quality of life as well as professional satisfaction in health care providers. A better understanding may also aid in the development of an educational framework that targets resources to better manage the innate stressors associated with caretaking.

VETERINARIANS AND MENTAL HEALTH

Veterinarians regularly face different forms of distress that may lead to feelings of burnout and compassion fatigue.[84] In 2014, a survey by the Centers for Disease Control and Prevention found that 1 in 6 veterinarians might have experienced suicidal ideation and that 1 in 11 may have serious psychological distress.[77] A stressful work environment in combination with an individual's lack of cognitive and emotional resources to engage in empathetic processing may contribute to an overall reduction in empathy.[58] Similarly, the inability to process and cope may further contribute to this decline. In veterinarians, it has been suggested that a diminished ability to escape into other outlets, and potentially adaptive ways of coping, such as the arts, literature, theater, or music, may negatively affect professional well-being.[34] Empathy in a clinical setting requires emotional agility as well as increased levels of self-regulation.[85,86]

Interestingly, veterinarians as a group may undervalue treatment of mental health conditions as well as have a more negative perception of the level of care those with mental illness receive.[77] Whether or not these findings affect veterinary medicine and its willingness to seek out resources regarding mental health remains unclear. Veterinary support groups that aim to promote sharing, livelihood, and conversations that foster empathy in the profession have been proposed.[34] Implementing focused training within veterinary curriculums, as well as beyond, might be an area of opportunity to lay a foundation for some of these tactics. Increasing awareness and conversations in the profession may reduce stigmas associated with self-care and may ultimately promote veterinarians to be in a stronger position to care for others. In addition, continued research into the concept of empathetic communication specifically, as opposed to discussion of feelings of empathy alone, may give veterinarians new insights as to how to improve client-patient relationships, as well as professional satisfaction.[19] Finally, a deeper understanding of medical culture, and how the institutional and economic factors that comprise it, may impede one's ability to provide empathetic health care requires further investigation.[19] A clearer understanding of the factors that contribute to empathetic decline in the field may ultimately provide specific strategies to mitigate these trends and their negative effects, such as compassion fatigue. Furthermore, a better understanding of how a client or patient's responsiveness to empathy is conveyed back to a health care provider may help these providers experience more meaningful work with greater satisfaction.[87]

SUMMARY

Practicing empathy is considered an essential part of being a skilled veterinarian. Opportunities where an expression of empathy are warranted are abundant and may be directed toward patients, clients, colleagues, or a combination. Despite what are often daily occurrences, the expression of empathy is a nontechnical competency that can often be overlooked educationally, which may have a large impact on both the veterinarian as well as their patient. Surprisingly, there are few resources to teach or assess empathy accurately. Furthermore, opportunities to teach this skill in most of the veterinary curricula or continuing education are equally uncommon. The alarming trends in veterinarians of empathetic depletion, personal distress, and compassion fatigue highlight the need for new insights, teaching modalities, and interventions. A proactive approach that aims to manage through awareness and training as well as the creation of readily available resources that promote mental health support and offer strategies in resilience and coping are warranted. Identifying specific areas that help to improve professional well-being and mental health have the potential to translate into less impact from signs of compassion fatigue, improved displays of clinical empathy, and ultimately an increase in positive outcomes for both patients and their providers.

DISCLOSURE

The author has nothing to disclose.

REFERENCES

1. Eby D. Empathy in general practice: its meaning for patients and doctors. Br J Gen Pract 2018;68(674):412–3.
2. May W. Maintaining empathy in medical education. Med Teach 2013;35(12):977–8.
3. Cunico L, Sartori R, Marognolli O, et al. Developing empathy in nursing students: a cohort longitudinal study. J Clin Nurs 2012;21(13–14):2016–25.
4. Finset A, Mjaaland TA. The medical consultation viewed as a value chain: a neurobehavioral approach to emotion regulation in doctor-patient interaction. Patient Educ Couns 2009;74(3):323–30.
5. Rakel DP, Hoeft TJ, Barrett BP, et al. Practitioner empathy and the duration of the common cold. Fam Med 2009;41(7):494–501.
6. Stewart M, Brown JB, Weston WW, et al. Patient-centered medicine. Thousand Oaks (CA): Sage; 1995.
7. Greenhalgh T, Eversley J. Quality in general practice: towards a holistic approach. London: Kings Fund; 1999.
8. Association of American Medical Colleges. Report I: Learning objectives for medical student education—Guidelines for medical school. Acad Med 1999;74:13–8. Available at: http://journals.lww.com/academicmedicine/Abstract/1999/01001/Learning_objectives_for_medical_student.10.aspx.
9. Frank JR. The CanMEDS 2005 physician competency framework. Better standards. Better physicians. Better care. Ottawa (Canada): Royal College of Physicians and Surgeons of Canada; 2005.
10. Working Group Under a Mandate of the Joint Commission of the Swiss Medical Schools. Swiss Catalogue of Learning Objectives for Undergraduate Medical Training. Available at: http://sclo.smifk.ch.
11. Institute of Medicine. Crossing the quality chasm: a new health system for the 21st century. Washington, DC: National Academies Press; 2001.
12. Singer T, Klimecki OM. Empathy and compassion. Curr Biol 2014;24(18):R875–8.
13. Heyes C. Empathy is not in our genes. Neurosci Biobehav Rev 2018;95:499–507.
14. Svenaeus F. The phenomenology of empathy in medicine: an introduction. Med Health Care Philos 2014;17(2):245–8.

15. Weisz E, Zaki J. Motivated empathy: a social neuroscience perspective. Curr Opin Psychol 2018;24:67–71.
16. Baron-Cohen S. The science of evil: on empathy and the origins of cruelty. New York: Basic Books; 2011.
17. Kilner JM, Lemon RN. What we know currently about mirror neurons. Curr Biol 2013;23(23):R1057–62.
18. Coulehan JL, Platt FW, Egener B, et al. Let me see if i have this right...": words that help build empathy. Ann Intern Med 2001;135(3):221–7.
19. Halpern J. From idealized clinical empathy to empathic communication in medical care. Med Health Care Philos 2014;17(2):301–11.
20. Sinclair S, Beamer K, Hack TF, et al. Sympathy, empathy, and compassion: A grounded theory study of palliative care patients' understandings, experiences, and preferences. Palliat Med 2017;31(5):437–47.
21. Soanes C, Stevenson A. Compassion. In: Stevenson A, editor. Oxford English dictionary of English. 3rd edition. New York: Oxford University Press; 2010.
22. Soanes C, Stevenson A. Sympathy. In: Stevenson A, editor. Oxford English dictionary of English. 3rd edition. New York: Oxford University Press; 2010.
23. Soanes C, Stevenson A. Empathy. In: Stevenson A, editor. Oxford English dictionary of English. 3rd edition. New York: Oxford University Press; 2010.
24. Post SG, Ng LE, Fischel JE, et al. Routine, empathic and compassionate patient care: definitions, development, obstacles, education and beneficiaries. J Eval Clin Pract 2014;20(6):872–80.
25. Silverman J, Kurtz SA, Draper J. Skills for communicating with patients. Arbingdon, Oxfordshire, England: Radcliffe Medical Press; 2005.
26. Carson CA. Nonverbal communication in veterinary practice. Vet Clin North Am Small Anim Pract 2007;37(1):49–viii.
27. Brugel S, Postma-Nilsenová M, Tates K. The link between perception of clinical empathy and nonverbal behavior: The effect of a doctor's gaze and body orientation. Patient Educ Couns 2015;98(10):1260–5.
28. Lorié Á, Reinero DA, Phillips M, et al. Culture and nonverbal expressions of empathy in clinical settings: A systematic review. Patient Educ Couns 2017; 100(3):411–24.
29. Beck RS, Daughtridge R, Sloane PD. Physician-patient communication in the primary care office: a systematic review. J Am Board Fam Pract 2002;15(1):25–38.
30. Finset A, Piccolo LD. Nonverbal communication in clinical contexts. In: Rimondini M, editor. Communication in cognitive behavioral therapy. Springer Science + Business Media; 2011. p. 107–28. https://doi.org/10.1007/978-1-4419-6807-4_5.
31. Roter DL, Frankel RM, Hall JA, et al. The expression of emotion through nonverbal behavior in medical visits. Mechanisms and outcomes. J Gen Intern Med 2006; 21(Suppl 1):S28–34.
32. Ickes W, Stinson L, Bissonnette V, et al. Naturalistic social cognition: Empathic accuracy in mixed-sex dyads. J Pers Soc Psychol 1990;59(4):730–42.
33. Ickes W. Empathetic accuracy. New York City: Guilford Press; 1997.
34. Schoenfeld-Tacher RM, Kogan LR, Meyer-Parsons B, et al. Educational Research Report: Changes in Students' Levels of Empathy during the Didactic Portion of a Veterinary Program. J Vet Med Educ 2015;42(3):194–205.
35. Sulzer SH, Feinstein NW, Wendland CL. Assessing empathy development in medical education: a systematic review. Med Educ 2016;50(3):300–10.
36. Di Blasi Z, Harkness E, Ernst E, et al. Influence of context effects on health outcomes: a systematic review. Lancet 2001;357(9258):757–62.

37. Colliver JA, Conlee MJ, Verhulst SJ, et al. Reports of the decline of empathy during medical education are greatly exaggerated: a reexamination of the research. Acad Med 2010;85(4):588–93.
38. Hermans L, Olde Hartman TC, Dielissen PW. Differences between GP perception of delivered empathy and patient-perceived empathy: a cross-sectional study in primary care. Br J Gen Pract 2018;68(674):e621–6.
39. Hall JA, Stein TS, Roter DL, et al. Inaccuracies in physicians' perceptions of their patients. Med Care 1999;37(11):1164–8.
40. Mercer SW, Reynolds WJ. Empathy and quality of care. Br J Gen Pract 2002; 52(Suppl):S9–12.
41. Mercer SW, Maxwell M, Heaney D, et al. The consultation and relational empathy (CARE) measure: development and preliminary validation and reliability of an empathy-based consultation process measure. Fam Pract 2004;21(6):699–705.
42. Olson K, Kemper KJ. Factors associated with well-being and confidence in providing compassionate care. J Evid Based Complement Altern Med 2014; 19(4):292–6.
43. Ogle J, Bushnell JA, Caputi P. Empathy is related to clinical competence in medical care. Med Educ 2013;47(8):824–31.
44. Austin EJ, Evans P, Magnus B, et al. A preliminary study of empathy, emotional intelligence and examination performance in MBChB students. Med Educ 2007;41(7):684–9.
45. Ong LM, Visser MR, Lammes FB, et al. Doctor-patient communication and cancer patients' quality of life and satisfaction. Patient Educ Couns 2000;41(2):145–56.
46. Graugaard PK, Holgersen K, Finset A. Communicating with alexithymic and non-alexithymic patients: an experimental study of the effect of psychosocial communication and empathy on patient satisfaction. Psychother Psychosom 2004;73(2): 92–100.
47. Goodchild CE, Skinner TC, Parkin T. The value of empathy in dietetic consultations. A pilot study to investigate its effect on satisfaction, autonomy and agreement. J Hum Nutr Diet 2005;18(3):181–5.
48. Bertakis KD, Roter D, Putnam SM. The relationship of physician medical interview style to patient satisfaction. J Fam Pract 1991;32(2):175–81.
49. Stewart MA. Effective physician-patient communication and health outcomes: a review. CMAJ 1995 May 1;152(9):1423–33.
50. Jay S, Litt IF, Durant RH. Compliance with therapeutic regimens. J Adolesc Health Care 1984;5(2):124–36.
51. Maguire P, Faulkner A, Booth K, et al. Helping cancer patients disclose their concerns. Eur J Cancer 1996;32A(1):78–81.
52. Neumann M, Edelhäuser F, Tauschel D, et al. Empathy decline and its reasons: a systematic review of studies with medical students and residents. Acad Med 2011 Aug;86(8):996–1009.
53. Kanji N, Coe JB, Adams CL, et al. Effect of veterinarian-client-patient interactions on client adherence to dentistry and surgery recommendations in companion-animal practice. J Am Vet Med Assoc 2012;240(4):427–36.
54. McArthur ML, Fitzgerald JR. Companion animal veterinarians' use of clinical communication skills. Aust Vet J 2013;91(9):374–80.
55. Lamm C, Batson CD, Decety J. The neural substrate of human empathy: effects of perspective-taking and cognitive appraisal. J Cogn Neurosci 2007 Jan;19(1): 42–58.
56. Did you know? Compassion Fatigue Awareness Project. Available at: http://compassionfatigue.org/. Accessed February 11, 2021.

57. Cohen SP. Compassion fatigue and the veterinary health team. Vet Clin North Am Small Anim Pract 2007;37(1):123–ix.

58. Gleichgerrcht E, Decety J. Empathy in clinical practice: how individual dispositions, gender, and experience moderate empathic concern, burnout, and emotional distress in physicians. PLoS One 2013;8(4):e61526.

59. Duarte J, Pinto-Gouveia J. Empathy and feelings of guilt experienced by nurses: A cross-sectional study of their role in burnout and compassion fatigue symptoms. Appl Nurs Res 2017;35:42–7.

60. Decety J, Lamm C. Empathy versus personal distress: Recent evidence from social neuroscience. In: Decety J, Ickes W, editors. Social neuroscience. The social neuroscience of empathy. MIT Press; 2009. p. 199–213. https://doi.org/10.7551/mitpress/9780262012973.003.0016.

61. Hunt P, Denieffe S, Gooney M. Running on empathy: Relationship of empathy to compassion satisfaction and compassion fatigue in cancer healthcare professionals. Eur J Cancer Care (Engl) 2019;28(5):e13124.

62. Hojat M, Vergare MJ, Maxwell K, et al. The devil is in the third year: a longitudinal study of erosion of empathy in medical school [published correction appears in Acad Med. 2009 Nov;84(11):1616]. Acad Med 2009;84(9):1182–91.

63. Hojat M, Mangione S, Nasca TJ, et al. An empirical study of decline in empathy in medical school. Med Educ 2004;38(9):934–41.

64. Newton BW, Barber L, Clardy J, et al. Is there hardening of the heart during medical school? Acad Med 2008;83(3):244–9.

65. Bellini LM, Baime M, Shea JA. Variation of mood and empathy during internship. JAMA 2002;287(23):3143–6.

66. Bellini LM, Shea JA. Mood change and empathy decline persist during three years of internal medicine training. Acad Med 2005;80(2):164–7.

67. West CP, Huschka MM, Novotny PJ, et al. Association of perceived medical errors with resident distress and empathy: a prospective longitudinal study. JAMA 2006;296(9):1071–8.

68. West CP, Huntington JL, Huschka MM, et al. A prospective study of the relationship between medical knowledge and professionalism among internal medicine residents. Acad Med 2007;82(6):587–92.

69. Rosen IM, Gimotty PA, Shea JA, et al. Evolution of sleep quantity, sleep deprivation, mood disturbances, empathy, and burnout among interns. Acad Med 2006;81(1):82–5.

70. Shaw JR, Adams CL, Bonnett BN, et al. Use of the roter interaction analysis system to analyze veterinarian-client-patient communication in companion animal practice. J Am Vet Med Assoc 2004;225(2):222–9.

71. Chen D, Lew R, Hershman W, et al. A cross-sectional measurement of medical student empathy. J Gen Intern Med 2007;22(10):1434–8.

72. Thomas MR, Dyrbye LN, Huntington JL, et al. How do distress and well-being relate to medical student empathy? A multicenter study. J Gen Intern Med 2007;22(2):177–83.

73. Stratton TD, Saunders JA, Elam CL. Changes in medical students' emotional intelligence: an exploratory study. Teach Learn Med 2008;20(3):279–84.

74. Hogeveen J, Salvi C, Grafman J. 'Emotional Intelligence': Lessons from Lesions. Trends Neurosci 2016;39(10):694–705.

75. Adin DB, Royal KD, Adin CA. Cross-Sectional Assessment of the Emotional Intelligence of Fourth-Year Veterinary Students and Veterinary House Officers in a Teaching Hospital. J Vet Med Educ 2020;47(2):193–201.

76. Nunes P, Williams S, Sar B, et al. A study of empathy decline in students from five health disciplines during their first year of training. Int J Med Educ 2011;2:12–7.
77. Nett RJ, Witte TK, Holzbauer SM, et al. Risk factors for suicide, attitudes toward mental illness, and practice-related stressors among US veterinarians. J Am Vet Med Assoc 2015;247(8):945–55.
78. Arbe Montoya AI, Hazel S, Matthew SM, et al. Moral distress in veterinarians. Vet Rec 2019;185(20):631.
79. O'Connor E. Sources of work stress in veterinary practice in the UK. Vet Rec 2019;184(19):588.
80. Dawson BF, Thompson NJ. The Effect of Personality on Occupational Stress in Veterinary Surgeons. J Vet Med Educ 2017;44(1):72–83.
81. Hafen M Jr, Reisbig AM, White MB, et al. Predictors of depression and anxiety in first-year veterinary students: a preliminary report. J Vet Med Educ 2006;33(3):432–40.
82. Hafen M Jr, Ratcliffe GC, Rush BR. Veterinary medical student well-being: depression, stress, and personal relationships. J Vet Med Educ 2013;40(3):296–302.
83. Siqueira Drake AA, Hafen M Jr, Rush BR, et al. Predictors of anxiety and depression in veterinary medicine students: a four-year cohort examination. J Vet Med Educ 2012;39(4):322–30.
84. Moses L, Malowney MJ, Wesley Boyd J. Ethical conflict and moral distress in veterinary practice: A survey of North American veterinarians. J Vet Intern Med 2018;32(6):2115–22.
85. Decety J, Jackson PL. The functional architecture of human empathy. Behav Cogn Neurosci Rev 2004;3(2):71–100.
86. Dewall CN, Baumeister RF, Gailliot MT, et al. Depletion makes the heart grow less helpful: helping as a function of self-regulatory energy and genetic relatedness. Pers Soc Psychol Bull 2008;34(12):1653–62.
87. Shanafelt TD, West C, Zhao X, et al. Relationship between increased personal well-being and enhanced empathy among internal medicine residents. J Gen Intern Med 2005;20(7):559–64.

Suicide Warning Signs and What to Do

Christine Moutier, MD, Maggie G. Mortali, MPH*

KEYWORDS

- Suicide/suicide prevention • Suicide risk factors • Suicide warning signs
- Protective factors • Mental health • Depression • Resilience

KEY POINTS

- Suicide is a complex health outcome with multiple intersecting risk and protective factors.
- Critical to suicide prevention is helping the person connect with hope and reasons for living while at the same time, helping them feel less connected to reasons for wanting to die.
- Key features of suicide prevention initiatives for veterinary professionals include reducing stigma associated with mental health distress and help seeking, improving access to peer or social support and to health care, and making judicious changes related to access to lethal means in the professional work setting.

INTRODUCTION

Suicide is a major public health problem worldwide with approximately 800,000 people dying by suicide each year.[1] In the United States, suicide is the 10th leading cause of death with the loss of more than 47,000 Americans to suicide in 2019.[2] Suicide has a devastating impact on individuals, family, friends, colleagues, and communities. Suicide affects every demographic and occupational group, but some groups may be at higher risk than others. Research has shown that the suicide rate among veterinarians is higher than that of the general population.[3] According to a 2019 study of suicide among veterinarians in the United States from 1979 through 2015, researchers used records of deceased US veterinarians and found that, compared with the general US population, male veterinarians were 2.1 times and female veterinarians were 3.5 times as likely to die by suicide as their gender-matched controls in the general population.[3] During this era of the pandemic and even before it, attitudes toward mental health and mental health care have been opening up tremendously,[4] and science demonstrates that suicide, although complex, is a health issue and a generally

American Foundation for Suicide Prevention, 199 Water Street, Floor 11, New York, NY 10038, USA
* Corresponding author.
E-mail address: mmortali@afsp.org
Twitter: @cmoutierMD (C.M.); @MaggieAFSP (M.G.M.)

Vet Clin Small Anim 51 (2021) 1053–1060
https://doi.org/10.1016/j.cvsm.2021.04.021

preventable cause of death. Therefore, implementing steps to prevent suicide among veterinary professionals can drive down the suicide rate and save lives.

SUICIDE RISK FACTORS

There is no single cause for suicide. Rather there are multiple, intersecting factors that come together to create suicide risk. Suicide risk factors are characteristics or conditions that increase the chance a person may take their life. Suicide most often occurs when stressors and health issues converge to create an experience of hopelessness and despair. As with most health outcomes, individual factors dynamically interact with environmental factors to impact individual mental health and suicide risk. Similar to a person who is at risk for heart disease due to high blood pressure, or a family history of heart disease, some people are at higher risk for suicide than others.

Suicide Risk Factors: Biological Factors

Biological factors most significant to suicide risk include mental health conditions.[4,5] Research has shown that 85% to 95% of people who die by suicide have a diagnosable mental health condition at the time of their death.[6] Depression is by far the most common mental health condition in general and is the one that most commonly increases suicide risk.[7] According to the 2019 National Survey on Drug Use and Health, approximately 51.5 million adults aged 18 years or older (20.6% of all US adults) experienced a mental health condition, with 13.1 million adults aged 18 years or older (5.2% of all US adults) having experienced a serious mental illness within the past year.[8] In a 2014 convenience sample survey of more than 11,000 US veterinarians, 9% reported current serious psychological distress and 31% reported experiencing depressive episodes since leaving veterinary school, each more prevalent than in the general population.[9] Regional surveys of US veterinarians showed similar findings, reporting higher levels of anxiety, depression, and compassion fatigue among veterinarians, compared with the general populations of the same regions.[10–15]

Despite the prevalence of mental health conditions and suicide risk among adults, approximately two-thirds of individuals with symptoms meeting clinical criteria for mental and substance use disorders do not receive treatment.[16] There are several reasons people do not seek treatment. Professionals with mental health conditions often face work-related discrimination or fear such discrimination, fears such as limits on independence, increase in supervision, jeopardized job security, or restriction of their career advancement. This fear often results in individuals taking great lengths to ensure that coworkers and managers do not find out about their mental health conditions, which includes avoiding employee assistance programs and effective treatment options.

Physical health conditions are also known to contribute to suicide risk, most often when they co-occur with depression, anxiety, substance use disorders, or other mental health conditions. For example, studies show that many chronic conditions such as chronic pain, heart disease, chronic pulmonary disease, traumatic brain injury, and human immunodeficiency virus/AIDS significantly increase suicide risk.[17] These serious health conditions are not thought to elevate suicide risk in isolation, but rather contribute to suicide risk in combination with other suicide risk factors.

Suicide Risk Factors: Psychological Factors

Particular psychological risk factors are also known to increase suicide risk. As with health-related or biological risk factors, it is not any of these on their own, but rather in combination with other risk factors or life events, that increase an individual's risk for suicide. Individuals who have problems with decision making, problem solving, and other cognitive functions, for example, are shown to be at a higher risk for suicide. Note that an individual's inability to tolerate conflict is not a sign of potential suicide risk when considered in isolation. And high driving perfectionism similarly can be adaptive in many ways toward functioning and fulfilling career and other life roles. However, these psychological traits can potentially contribute to suicide risk when they intersect with other risk factors and stressors, such as a current major depressive episode or a personal or professional setback or loss. Psychological factors often intensify an individual's negative perceptions and feelings in reaction to stressful life events and interpersonal interactions. These risk factors may decrease an individual's ability to solve problems or seek help and can increase the likelihood of responding impulsively rather than mindfully considering many options to approach about a challenging situation.

Psychological risk factors can also include psychological experiences that increase the short-term risk for suicide. Periods of transition in a person's life often trigger new or latent psychological shifts, which can exacerbate suicide risk in those with underlying risk. For some individuals, the psychological impact of transitions in relationship status, occupation, or financial status can diminish one's resilience reserve, which can lead to greater negative impact of other risk factors on mental health and coping, which in turn can lead to a sense of hopelessness and worthlessness that can increase suicide risk. Similarly, individuals experiencing shame and humiliation related to a current stressor, for example, legal or work related, can provide a sense of failure, rejection, and disconnection from their support network.

Suicide Risk Factors: Social and Environmental Factors

Social and environmental factors (and current factors such as bullying, relationship, and financial or cultural factors) also contribute as risk factors for suicide. Social and environmental factors can also be job related, such as isolated or demanding occupations, stressful work environments, and work-home imbalance. Any prolonged stress, including harassment, workplace bullying, relationship problems, legal problems, and unemployment, can also serve as social/environmental risk factors. Perhaps one of the most significant environmental risk factors is access to a method for killing oneself, which is referred to as access to lethal means.

In a study of death records for more than 11,000 US veterinarians over a 36-year period, the use of firearms was the most common method among the 398 suicide decedents, which is also true for general population suicide decedents. Notably, 39% of suicide deaths among veterinarians were the result of pharmaceutical poisoning, a rate nearly 2.5 times that for individuals in the general US population.[3] Research shows that individuals at risk for suicide often use methods that are accessible and familiar to them,[18–20] and veterinarians have access to and knowledge of lethal pharmaceutical products.[21,22] Every type of lethal means that has been studied has found similar results: when you limit access to lethal means, suicide risk decreases. This fact is true for methods including the detoxification of the domestic gas supply in the United Kingdom, bans on toxic pesticides in Sri Lanka, and decreases in household firearm ownership in the United States, in which all were followed by significant reductions in method-specific suicides as well as overall suicide rates in these countries.[23]

The combination of biological, psychological, social, and environmental risk factors all contributes to an individual's risk for suicide. For example, a person who loses their job (social/environmental) and job-centered identity and self-worth (psychological) may also be experiencing a mental health condition (biological plus). Therefore, this person may see no way out of the situation. These factors can come together to lead to hopelessness and a lack of problem solving or hope for the future. This, combined with prolonged occupational stress, paired with access to lethal means, creates a high-risk situation for suicide.

SUICIDE WARNING SIGNS

Suicide risk factors often endure over a long period, whereas suicide warning signs can signal more imminent suicidal risk.

Suicide Warning Signs: Talk

Individuals who are thinking about suicide often talk about ending their lives directly or indirectly. Some people may make their intentions known by saying they have no reason to live or would be better off dead, whereas other people may be less direct and say they feel trapped or are in unbearable pain. Some individuals may only hint at their feelings of despair, and these types of comments may be subtle, even laced with humor, and often can go unnoticed. It is important to take what a person says seriously, especially when displaying other suicide warning signs.

Suicide Warning Signs: Behavior

Behaviors that may signal risk, especially if related to a painful event, loss, or significant change, can include an increased use of alcohol or drugs; withdrawing from activities and/or isolating from family, friends, and coworkers; or looking for a way to end their life, such as searching for methods. Additional warning signs related to a person's behavior may involve absences from work, which can include being late for work or for meetings and appointments, leaving work early, and/or taking more sick days than usual. There also may be a noticeable shift in a person's typical work performance, which can include missing deadlines, decline in quality of work, or being agitated or easily distracted.

Suicide Warning Signs: Mood

We all have ups and downs in our mood, so when it comes to warning signs for suicide, it is important to look for changes that seem uncharacteristic or concerning. For example, if a person has struggled with depression, mood changes can signal mental health symptoms are worsening and risk is increasing. Another example could be something sudden, such as unexplained happiness in someone who has been depressed, which can indicate that the individual has decided on a plan and is relieved he or she will no longer be in pain. Although warning signs are not always obvious, understanding suicide warning signs can help you recognize when someone is at an increased risk (**Table 1**).

WHAT YOU CAN DO

Suicide, although complex, is a health issue. Therefore, it is important that we all do our part in approaching mental health and suicide risk in a similar manner to other health issues. Individuals should be able to receive support and access to care to have their mental health needs addressed. Just as with physical health concerns, people can choose how and who is involved with their mental health. The more proactive we are, prioritizing our own mental health and discussing mental health in appropriate ways in the workplace arena, the more we can contribute to a culture of safety and respect, in which individuals understand that it is safe to receive mental health care when they need it.

Table 1
Suicide warning signs

Talk	Behavior	Mood
A person showing signs of suicide risk may talk about: • Killing themself • Feeling hopeless • Being a burden to others • Feeling trapped • Being in unbearable pain	Behaviors that may signal risk include: • Increased use of alcohol or drugs • Looking for a way to end one's life • Withdrawing from activities • Isolating from family/friends •Sleeping too much or too little • Visiting/calling people to say goodbye • Giving away prized possessions • Aggression • Fatigue	People at risk for suicide can display any of the following moods: • Depressed • Anxious • Loss of interest • Irritability • Humiliation or shame • Agitation or anger • Relief or sudden improvement

It is important to note that distress leads many people to instinctually withdraw, just at a time when receiving support is even more important. In addition, workplace cultures that traditionally emphasize self-sufficiency or stoicism may unintentionally create additional barriers to reaching out for help. Therefore, many people who experience suicidal thoughts do not disclose them to anyone. If someone does mention they are struggling in the aforementioned ways, you can thank them for opening up and let them know you want to support them, and that you are there to help them find the help they need.

A person in a mental health crisis or at risk for suicide may not reach out and ask for help directly, but that does not mean that help is not wanted. Most people who are suicidal are ambivalent about taking their life and really just want relief to their pain: part of them wants to live and part of them wants to die. Critical to suicide prevention is helping the person connect with hope and reasons for living while at the same time, helping them feel less connected to reasons for wanting to die. If you think someone you know is thinking about suicide, assume you are the only one who will reach out. Having an honest conversation with the person will let them know that you care. Ask directly if they are thinking about suicide. Take the person seriously and speak up if you are concerned about them. Help the person by connecting with crisis resources and services immediately. The following are some tips for talking with someone who may be experiencing a mental health crisis or who may be at risk for suicide.

1. Engage the person in a private one-to-one conversation and let them know you are concerned, what you have observed, and that you are there only to support them. Ask open-ended questions and enquire about how they are doing,

2. Let the person know you are listening. Reassure the person that you hear what they are saying and that you are taking what they say seriously. For example, "I'm so glad you're telling me about how much has been going on, and how you're feeling. Thank you for sharing this with me."

3. Show the person your support. In your own way, make sure the person knows that you are there with them, and that you care. Encourage the person to continue talking and really listen to what they are saying. Let the person know that you want to hear more about how they are feeling and what they are going through.

4. Ask the person about changes in their life and how they are coping. Find out how long the person has been feeling this way and any changes these feelings or circumstances have caused in their life. For example, "How long have you felt this way?" or, "Can you share more about when these feelings started?"

5. If you suspect, even slightly, that the person is thinking about suicide, trust your gut and ask them directly. For example, "Sometimes when people are feeling this way, they have thoughts about ending their life. Are you thinking about killing yourself?" or, "Are you having thoughts about suicide?" Research shows that asking a person about suicide will not put the idea or thoughts about suicide in their head, rather the person will most likely be relieved that someone cares enough to hear about their experience with suicidal thoughts.[24,25] It is important to not come off like you are passing judgment. For example, do not say, "You're not thinking of doing something stupid, are you?" or guilt-trip them by saying, "Think of what it would do to your family." Instead, reassure the person that you understand and care.

6. If the person tells you they are thinking about suicide, stay calm. It is important to remember that just because someone is having thoughts of suicide that does not mean they are in immediate danger. Take the time to calmly listen to what they have to say and ask some follow-up questions: "How often are you having these thoughts?" or "What do you need to do to feel safe?" Reassure the person that help is available and that these feelings are a signal that it is time to talk to a mental health professional. Follow their lead and know when to take a break. This is a tough conversation to have, so make sure the other person knows they can stop if it feels like talking about it is too hard for them at the moment.

   If the person you are talking with indicates they are thinking about suicide that is an indication they should speak with a health professional. For example, you can say, "I hear you that you're struggling, and I think it would really be helpful for you to talk to a professional who can help you" or "I really think talking to someone can help you gain some perspective and keep things from getting worse." You can reassure them that you will also continue to be there for them while they seek professional help.

7. Help the person connect with help. Sometimes making that first contact to professional help can be the hardest. Offer to help them connect in whatever way you are comfortable with. It is important to keep in mind that not everyone is ready right away. If the person refuses your suggestion of professional help (and if they are not in immediate danger, ie, that they are not presently self-harming or about to), be patient and do not push too hard. For example, "It's okay that it doesn't sound like you're ready yet. I really hope you'll think about it. Just let me know if you change your mind, and I can help you connect with someone" or "If you're not ready to go in and meet with someone in person, you could call the National Suicide Prevention Lifeline at 1-800-273-8255, or if you don't feel like speaking, just text TALK to the Crisis Text Line at 741741. They can tell you more about what it might be like to work with a doctor, counselor or therapist."

If the person is in immediate danger, stay with them and help to remove or secure all lethal means in their environment. Call the National Suicide Prevention Lifeline or the Crisis Text Line and encourage them to seek help or to contact a doctor or therapist.

SUMMARY

We can no longer accept as status quo that suicide rates are higher among veterinary professionals compared with the general population. Like the public's mounting interest in suicide prevention, the readiness within veterinary medicine to address suicide risk among its own is mounting and encouraging. Shedding stigma and prioritizing our own mental health, making access to mental health care a priority, and learning ways to support our colleagues are all ways to contribute to a culture that reduces suicide risk.

DISCLOSURE

The authors have nothing to disclose.

REFERENCES

1. World Health Organization (WHO). Suicide data. Available at: https://www.who. int/teams/mental-health-and-substance-use/suicide-data. Accessed February 9, 2021.
2. Centers for Disease Control and Prevention, National Centers for Injury Prevention and Control. Web-based Injury Statistics Query and Reporting System (WISQARS) [online]. Available at: www.cdc.gov/injury/wisqars. Accessed February 9, 2021.
3. Tomasi SE, Fechter-Leggett ED, Edwards NT, et al. Suicide among veterinarians in the United States from 1979 through 2015. J Am Vet Med Assoc 2019;254(1): 104–12.
4. PR Newswire. COVID-19 Reinforces A Renewed Call to Make Suicide Prevention a National Priority. 2020. Available at: https://www.prnewswire.com/news-releases/ covid-19-reinforces-a-renewed-call-to-make-suicide-prevention-a-national-priority-301121593.html. Accessed December 18, 2020.
5. Kessler RC, Borges G, Walters EE. Prevalence of and risk factors for lifetime suicide attempts in the National Comorbidity Survey. Arch Gen Psychiatry 1999; 56(7):617–26.
6. Nock MK, Borges G, Bromet EJ, et al. Cross-national prevalence and risk factors for suicidal ideation, plans and attempts. Br J Psychiatry 2008;192(2):98–105.
7. Cavanaugh JT, Carson AJ, Sharpe M, et al. Psychological autopsy studies of suicide: a systematic review. Psychol Med 2003;33(3):11.
8. Harris EC, Barraclough B. Suicide as an outcome for mental disorders. A meta-analysis. Br J Psychiatry 1997;170:23.
9. Substance Abuse and Mental Health Services Administration. Key substance use and mental health indicators in the United States: results from the 2019 National survey on drug Use and health (HHS Publication No. PEP20-07-01-001, NSDUH Series H-55). Rockville (MD): Center for Behavioral Health Statistics and Quality, Substance Abuse and Mental Health Services Administration; 2020. Available at: https://www.samhsa.gov/data/.
10. Nett RJ, Witte TK, Holzbauer SM, et al. Risk factors for suicide, attitudes toward mental illness, and practice-related stressors among US veterinarians. J Am Vet Med Assoc 2015;247:945–55, 955.
11. Fowler HN, Holzbauer SM, Smith KE, et al. Survey of occupational hazards in Minnesota veterinary practices in 2012. J Am Vet Med Assoc 2016;248:207–18.
12. Elkins AD, Kearney M. Professional burnout among female veterinarians in the United States. J Am Vet Med Assoc 1992;200:604–8.
13. Skipper GE, Williams JB. Failure to acknowledge high suicide risk among veterinarians. J Vet Med Educ 2012;39:79–82.
14. Han B, Crosby AE, Ortega LA, et al. Suicidal ideation, suicide attempt, and occupations among employed adults aged 18-64years in the United States. Compr Psychiatry 2016;66:176–86.
15. Stallones L, Doenges T, Dik BJ, et al. Occupation and suicide: Colorado, 2004–2006. Am J Ind Med 2013;56:1290–5.
16. Milner A, Spittal MJ, Pirkis J, et al. Suicide by occupation: systematic review and meta-analysis. Br J Psychiatry 2013;203:409–16.

17. Wang PS, Simon GE, Avorn J, et al. Telephone screening, outreach, and care management for depressed workers and impact on clinical and work productivity outcomes: a randomized controlled trial. JAMA 2007;298(12):1401–11.
18. Ahmedani BK, Peterson EL, Hu Y, et al. Major physical health conditions and risk of suicide. Am J Prev Med 2017;53(3):308–15.
19. Jones-Fairnie H, Ferroni P, Silburn S, et al. Suicide in Australian veterinarians. Aust Vet J 2008;86:114–6.
20. Mellanby RJ. Incidence of suicide in the veterinary profession in England and Wales. Vet Rec 2005;157:415–7.
21. Hawton K, Clements A, Simkin S, et al. Doctors who kill themselves: a study of the methods used for suicide. QJM 2000;93:351–7.
22. Bartram DJ, Baldwin DS. Veterinary surgeons and suicide: influences, opportunities and research directions. Vet Rec 2008;162:36–40.
23. Dawson BF, Thompson NJ. The effect of personality on occupational stress in veterinary surgeons. J Vet Med Educ 2017;44:72–83.
24. Gunnell D, Miller M. Strategies to prevent suicide. BMJ 2010;341:c3054.
25. Gould MS, Marrocco FA, Kleinman M, et al. Evaluating iatrogenic risk of youth suicide screening programs: a randomized controlled trial. JAMA 2005;293(13):1635–43.

Addressing Unsatisfactory Performance in Employees

Christopher A. Adin, DVM, DACVS

KEYWORDS

- Performance • Evaluation • Feedback • Veterinary • Multilevel

KEY POINTS

- Quality performance evaluations that are tied to tangible rewards contribute to increased productivity and enhanced employee satisfaction.
- Evaluations should contain data related to clinical performance, combined with multilevel feedback from clients, technicians, peers, and supervisors.
- Performance feedback should occur regularly (not only when there is a problem) so that positive feedback is intermixed with constructive comments.
- Do not sugarcoat and expect change; feedback must be direct and specific to be effective.
- Employees rarely self-correct; you will need to intervene quickly once a problem is recognized.

INTRODUCTION

All veterinarians are leaders of a team. If you have assumed an official administrative role in your practice, then providing feedback and performance evaluation is one of your job duties. Whether you seek these administrative roles or not, every veterinarian in small animal practice leads a team of technical and clerical staff with a common goal of providing excellent client service and patient care. Chances are, you are currently working with someone who is failing to perform their duties in a way that meets your expectations. However, you do not enjoy talking to employees about their unsatisfactory performance, so you are sugarcoating any feedback that you give, or you are bottling it up for weeks or months, until you lose your patience and snap. As a leader it is your responsibility to remedy this situation, because *it is extremely rare for someone to self-correct a performance issue*. This article helps to provide you with the tools to deliver appropriate and timely performance counseling to your employees and coworkers.

DETERRENTS TO PROVIDING PERFORMANCE FEEDBACK

Veterinarians are reluctant to provide performance feedback to their staff for a variety of reasons. First, clinicians may believe that they do not have the authority to perform

Department of Small Animal Clinical Sciences, University of Florida, Gainesville, FL, USA
E-mail address: adinc@ufl.edu

Vet Clin Small Anim 51 (2021) 1061–1069
https://doi.org/10.1016/j.cvsm.2021.04.022   vetsmall.theclinics.com

evaluations within their workplace. Smaller practices often lack a formal mechanism for performance evaluation or the standards for performance are not clearly articulated by the practice owner. One of the key steps to alleviating the anxiety associated with performance evaluations is to establish a clear infrastructure in your practice, stating who does the evaluations, when they are to happen, and articulating clear performance standards and mechanisms for advancement. Lastly, veterinarians may lack the training and experience in providing effective feedback, making them even more reluctant to risk those difficult conversations. Veterinarians need to embrace their position as leaders in the practice and take responsibility for maintaining the quality of the work environment and retaining good employees. Evidence suggests that regular, high-quality feedback leads to increased performance and increased satisfaction in health care workers.[1–5]

ISSUE SPOTTING

Human resource professionals know that timing is everything. Performance and behavioral issues must be identified and addressed early to minimize damage to workplace and to increase the likelihood of successful resolution. Performance problems that are overlooked can become incredibly difficult to deal with once they are ingrained and can have widespread impact on the workplace that simply cannot be reversed. High-performing technicians, receptionists, and veterinarians will leave your practice when they are subjected to mistreatment by a single bad actor, especially when they see that the supervisor is unwilling or unable to take the steps needed to change the situation. Thus, one of the key points in managing employees is to be watching for issues and to address them *immediately*, before it is too late.

DIAGNOSING THE PROBLEM

As with any affliction, we must diagnose the cause of performance problems before we can treat the disease and assist an employee in developing a performance improvement plan. In his book *Chairing the Academic Department, Leadership Among Peers*,[6] Allan Tucker describes that performance problems are typically related to either *personal* or *environmental* factors as listed in **Table 1**. Interestingly, this framework aligns perfectly with data from tens of thousands of workers in the United States, as outlined by Marcus Buckingham and Curt Coffman in their book: *First Break All the Rules: What the Greatest Managers Do Differently*.[7] In their analysis, Buckingham and Coffman identify factors that predict whether an employee will be retained in their current position. Insights from these experts can be helpful in determining the causes of unsatisfactory performance in both veterinarians and staff, as described below.

Table 1
Causes of poor performance in employees

Employee Problems	Environmental Problems
• Lack of competence	• Lack of integration into team
• Physical or mental inability to carry out duties	• Lack of incentives
• Lack of understanding of expectations	• Poor leadership
• Low emotional intelligence or poor communication skills	• Inadequate facilities or equipment

Modified from Allan Tucker's Chairing the Academic Department, Leadership Among Peers, pp 246-261.[6]

Employee Problems

Abilities and skills

An employee's work ability (their physical and psychological capacity to manage job duties) and their perceptions of self-efficacy have been shown to have significant effects on work engagement and psychological distress.[8] As exemplified in the aforementioned questions, some of the causes of unsatisfactory performance in employees can be remedied through targeted interventions. For example, a technician lacking information in key areas of knowledge or skills (eg, anesthesia drug dose calculations, drug interactions) can be augmented through provision of training, software apps, and coaching. Equipment can be provided that will help with work quality (eg, anesthesia monitoring equipment, access to gloves for patient handling). When mistakes are due to an employee's unawareness of performance expectations, clear articulation of workplace standards can be very helpful (eg, technicians must be at work to begin treatments at 7 AM; vacation days must be scheduled at least 1 week in advance). Other employee-related problems, such as physical inability to complete duties or a lack of talent in organizing complicated schedules, may require reassignment to a position that is more aligned with the person's capabilities and strengths. A leader must work to quickly identify the cause of poor performance, institute a plan for improvement, and provide adequate support. When this fails to achieve the desired outcome, it is time to assist that employee in moving on to another role.

Environmental Problems

Veterinarians and staff performance can be negatively affected by several external factors that must be recognized and corrected. Environmental factors will typically affect multiple members of the staff and cause widespread performance and retention issues in a practice. Importantly, responsibility for correcting these environmental factors falls on the practice manager or medical director.

Lack of Incentives

Across all industries, performance incentives have proved to be a necessary ingredient to encourage certain behaviors. Performance in physicians has been tied to financial incentives for decades and has proved to be an effective way to provide positive incentives for performance improvement.[9,10] A large study involving more than 10,000 German workers showed that performance appraisals without the potential for tangible benefits (bonuses, promotions) can actually be detrimental to employee morale and job satisfaction.[11] Incentives should be based on measures that extend beyond productivity and should reward employees who have advanced their skills, shown exceptional effort, and manifested collegiality and professionalism in communications.

Poor Leadership

Managers must establish credibility by modeling the integrity and performance that is expected of employees. A longitudinal study involving more than 400 workers showed that employee's perception of the leader's alignment with ideal leadership characteristics significantly affected their attitudes and well-being.[12] The interaction between the leader and the employee is a relationship and must involve mutual respect for feedback to be delivered and received in an effective manner. In their book *First, Break All the Rules*,[7] Buckingham and Coffman present data from Gallup surveys of tens of thousands of employees, showing that the direct supervisor is the most important determinant of employee retention and happiness. In particular, their data showed the power of positive feedback delivered regularly by middle management. High-performing employees who had received thanks and recognition for their contributions within the last 7 days were more likely to be retained.[7] On the contrary, high-performing employees who were exposed to uncorrected negative behaviors by colleagues were less likely to be retained.

MEASURING PERFORMANCE

Performance assessments must be accurate and credible to be effective; therefore, supervisors must have a system to collect accurate information as part of any evaluation.[4] Use of multisource data is essential in the health care industry and is an evidence-based approach to measuring performance. Physician performance data derived from peers, supervisors, patients, and self have been shown to have high reliability ratings and are independent, with each providing unique information to the recipient.[13] Several "360°" survey instruments have been developed, allowing veterinary and human hospitals to obtain quality multisource feedback in a consistent manner for physicians, veterinarians, and administrators.[1,14] Initially, health care employees were evaluated only by people from within their own profession[15]; however, patient and client surveys began to be incorporated in the late 1990s and are now regularly used in large hospitals throughout the world.[16] Client feedback can be obtained using validated survey instruments at the time of discharge, such as the Communication Assessment Tool,[17] though client-sourced feedback tends to lack specific suggestions for improvement.[17] Our large academic veterinary hospital uses patient satisfaction surveys as part of the overall quality assessment program. Some of the more technical aspects of physician performance can be effectively evaluated by comparison of patient level outcomes derived from examining medical records, providing that those outcome measures are well tested.[9] In any hospital, performance data should be compared with the mean values for the unit and the organization, so that the effects of the work environment can be considered (eg, if all patient satisfaction scores are low, this may be an institutional problem and not an individual performance problem).

FREQUENCY AND FORMAT OF EVALUATIONS

Most of the private and academic veterinary practices provide formal feedback through annual evaluations, which are tied to merit- or production-based raises and to renewal of contracts. Tying tangible rewards with evaluations has been shown to increase acceptance by employees[11]; however, feedback is more effective in changing behaviors when it is given shortly after an event, occurring as often as once per week.[18] In fact, a recent study showed that timing outweighed specificity of the feedback, meaning that even global feedback provided regularly may be more effective than specific feedback provided long after an event.[18] It is important to avoid providing feedback on performance only when correction is needed, taking opportunities to call out specific positive behaviors when things are going well. Thus, a best-practices approach would combine frequent, lower stakes performance "check-ins" and coaching, followed by a formal annual evaluation, which is tied to tangible monetary rewards (merit raises or bonuses) and promotions. Although it is often convenient to deliver feedback electronically (via email or text), this is never the best method for constructive feedback. Specific recommendations for each methodology are described in the following section.

HOW TO DELIVER THE INFORMATION AND COUNSELING
Informal, Regular Feedback for Clinical Teams

Frequent discussion of performance in a small team can be carried out on a weekly basis, focusing on a review of goals at the beginning of the week (setting expectations), then debriefing and giving feedback at the end of the week. For example,

1. Monday morning, first thing: team huddle. The leader assembles the clinical team for a 5-minute discussion. Ask "What are we going to focus on this week?", develop a team consensus, and set clear goals with measurable outcomes. For example, "Tammy, I'd like you to focus on keeping our controlled drug logs up to date as you draw up each anesthetic dose. Bob, I'd like you to work on getting the prescriptions filled for our surgery discharges prior to the client's arrival-this has been a hold up lately and I know that we can be more efficient."
2. Friday afternoon: team febrief. The leader assembles the clinical team (or individual technician) for a 5-minute debrief. Have each team member comment on what went well and what could go better next time. As the leader, make sure to call out specific examples of good performance: "Tammy, great job keeping the controlled drug logs up to date this week-you have developed a great system that we can all learn from!" Where there is need for improvement, be specific and set expectations in a kind but clear manner: "Bob, we are still struggling to get those prescriptions for our surgery patients filled and at the front desk before the scheduled time of discharge. What can we do to make this work?"

Formal Annual Evaluation

Formal annual or semiannual evaluations using a standardized rubric and process should be a part of every veterinary practice's human resource system. An example of a clinical performance evaluation rubric is presented in **Fig. 1**. As previously discussed, formal evaluations should be associated with the potential for tangible rewards and should be based on data that are obtained from multilevel sources (clients, staff, peers, and supervisors) as well as productivity data related to the area of effort. Although a written evaluation document is essential, this should be accompanied by a face-to-face meeting with every employee, to enable the use of communications techniques described as follows:

Process for the meeting:

- Send out a rubric and ask the employee to complete a self-evaluation using the same system that you will use for your written evaluation (see example in **Fig. 1**).
- Schedule a meeting after receiving the employee's self-evaluation. Meet in an office or conference room with a closed door to ensure confidentiality. A mentor or employee advocate may be invited at the discretion of the employee, to provide support and additional input.
- At the beginning of the meeting, start a dialogue using open-ended questions, that do not have a "yes" or "no" answer, getting the employee involved in the conversation. Having the employee discuss their self-evaluation is an excellent way to start, and allows the supervisor to gain useful insights on the employee's awareness of any performance issues. For example,

I am really glad that we have this time to discuss your performance and your satisfaction with your job. You've had some time to reflect on the rubric and to perform your self-evaluation. Tell me how you think you have been doing this year.

- Make observations on areas that require improvement, then encourage employee involvement in the solutions by using open-ended questions. Be sure to use facts rather than subjective statements.

I noticed that you have been arriving after 8:00 in the mornings and I wondered what you thought was causing that to happen.

- Empathize and normalize, giving examples of how you or others have faced similar challenges.

That can be tough, I struggled with daycare options when my kids were young. How can we work out a way for you to get to work on time and still take care of your family in the morning? Do we need to work out a different schedule for you?

- Based on the information that you acquire through active enquiry, determine what the cause is, considering the personal and environmental factors outlined earlier in this article.
- Make a plan to remediate the problem and provide the necessary support to achieve that plan. Performance counseling that involves coaching and facilitation has been shown to be most effective.[4] The focus of coaching is getting the best performance out of the employee and involves positive psychology (I *will* do this), instead of dwelling on problems (I will *not* do that).
- For clinical performance, consider using "audit and feedback," a method that involves direct observation of clinical work or documentation of outcomes (client satisfaction, completion of medical records, adverse events, etc.), followed by delivery of specific feedback that focuses on achieving the desired outcomes. Audit and feedback were shown to be effective in improving clinical performance in 23 of 24 prospective studies, when feedback was delivered in both oral and written format, sourced from a colleague (not a supervisor), and includes specific targets and actions plans.[19]
- NOTE: end the meeting by stating your expectations clearly. Be direct and be specific; people will typically mince words here to avoid conflict, but you are setting yourself and the employee up for failure if you do not clearly express your expectations.

I expect you to arrive by 8:00 AM, dressed and prepared for work", NOT... "Please consider ways to improve your timeliness in the mornings so that we can get the day started on time.

- Follow-up the meeting by stating your expectations clearly, in writing. You can use an email to document this or better yet, a formal evaluation form.

UF VETERINARY HOSPITALS
FACULTY EVALUATION BY SERVICE CHIEF *of Clinical Performance*
Evaluation period: *January - December 2019*   **Evaluation due by January 26, 2020**

Faculty Evaluated:

Dr. Jim Shorts

Faculty Clinician Responsibilities Rating Scale: 1 = Unsatisfactory, 2 = Needs Improvement, 3 = Satisfactory, 4 = Strong, 5 = Superior, NA = Not Applicable

	1	2	3	4	5	N/A
1. Overall management of clinical cases	O	O	O	O	⊙	O
2. Use of state of the art or novel clinical techniques	O	O	O	O	⊙	O
3. Availability for cases, consultations, and transfers	O	O	O	⊙	O	O
4. Supervision and training of house officers	O	O	O	O	⊙	O
5. Supervision and training of veterinary students	O	O	O	O	⊙	O
6. Places the patient/client first	O	O	O	O	⊙	O
7. Provides estimates and client permission forms for surgery/anesthesia	O	O	O	O	⊙	O
8. Demonstrates professionalism, integrity, compassion, and trust	O	O	O	⊙	O	O
9. Communicates timely and effectively with clients and RDVMs	O	O	⊙	O	⊙	O
10. Communication is effective with all hospital personnel	O	O	O	⊙	O	O
11. Contributes to a culture of patient safety and continuous quality improvement	O	O	O	O	⊙	O
12. Familiarity with and adherence to hospital practices and policies	O	O	O	⊙	O	O

PLEASE RATE YOUR FACULTY MEMBER'S PERFORMANCE OVERALL
Rating Scale: 1 = Unsatisfactory, 2 = Needs Improvement, 3 = Satisfactory, 4 = Strong, 5 = Superior, NA = Not Applicable

	1	2	3	4	5	N/A
Overall Rating	O	O	O	⊙	O	O

Comments (Please include strengths and opportunities and areas for improvement)

Dr. Shorts has advanced the care of our patients through application of his skills in minimally invasive and laser surgery. Aside from the direct impact on caseload and revenue generation, the availability of these techniques has elevated the regional reputation of the practice in a way that is hard to quantify. His volunteer contributions to technician education and to visiting K-12 schools are great examples of his dedication to his profession and the practice.

Dr. Shorts and I have discussed that he needs to document his client communications in the medical record. Failure to include his phone and email conversations has led to loss of continuity for other staff that interact with the clients, inefficiency in finding information, and has even led to near misses regarding potential medication interactions as other clinicians prescribe medications for patients.

Faculty Signature	Service Chief Signature	CMO Signature	ADCS Signature

Fig. 1. A clinical performance evaluation form is presented, with a rubric and examples of specific performance feedback. (Used with permission from Dr. Dana Zimmel, University of Florida.)

- Make a plan to revisit the issue at predetermined time points in the future (1 month and 3 months) to assess progress. At each meeting document performance in writing, using facts and quantitiave information whenever possible.
- DO YOUR PART. In nearly every performance issue, the leader should be part of the solution, providing training where there are deficits, updating equipment or technology to facilitate the work, and making sure that expectations are clear. You are the leader, and ultimately, you share responsibility in the outcomes.

What to Do When "Plan A" Does not Work

In some instances, an employee will not be able to meet performance expectations, even with appropriate coaching. In these cases, documentation of the evaluations and the performance is of utmost importance. Employees should be placed on probation and provided with a performance improvement plan that has a well-defined

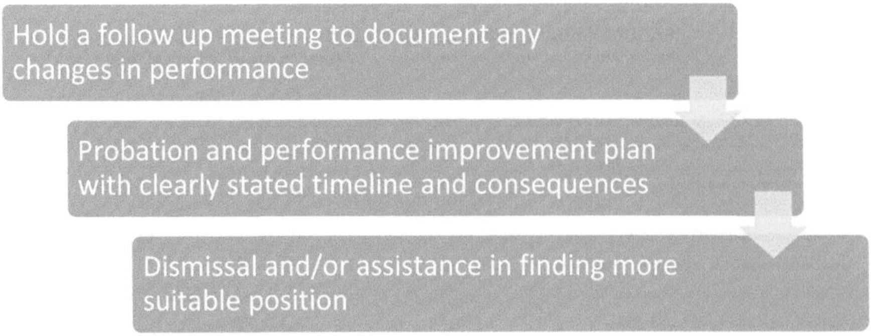

Hold a follow up meeting to document any changes in performance

Probation and performance improvement plan with clearly stated timeline and consequences

Dismissal and/or assistance in finding more suitable position

Fig. 2. When an employee fails to respond to specific performance feedback, a deliberate process should be followed that includes setting specific performance expectations, a probation period with a clear date for reassessment, documentation of failure to achieve the criteria, and a process for dismissal.

timeline and expected outcomes as depicted in **Fig. 2**. If an employee does not meet minimum performance requirements, even after being provided with counseling, training, and adequate support, it is time to discuss a change—moving on to another position that is more suited to their skills. When performed properly, termination of an employee can be paired with assistance in redirecting them toward an area of strength where they can be more satisfied with their own work over the remainder of their career.

Employee Relations Issues

Employees who practice bullying, harassment, yelling, throwing of instruments, harm patients in anger, or commit crimes are subject to quick and decisive action by the supervisor. A disciplinary process should be established in every practice for these "HR" violations, which is separate from the aforementioned formal evaluation process and can be enacted at any time during the evaluation cycle. Corrective actions should escalate with repeat offenses or can move directly to termination depending on the severity of the offense (a crime, for example). A typical progression for disciplinary action over time would be verbal warning, written reprimand, suspension without pay/demotion, and termination.

Confidentiality

Employers should maintain confidentiality regarding employee performance evaluations and any disciplinary actions. An employer who shares this information could be subject to defamation lawsuits by a disgruntled employee. Although maintaining confidentiality may seem simple, it can be difficult for a leader who is not allowed to tell a victim in the workplace what disciplinary action (if any) has been carried out after they have registered a complaint against an individual for unprofessional acts. Ultimately, this becomes a matter of trust; the employees must believe that the administrators in their practice will do the right thing, even when confidentiality prevents them from being transparent on some issues.

DISCLOSURE

The author has nothing to disclose.

REFERENCES

1. Hall W, Violato C, Lewkonia R, et al. Assessment of physician performance in Alberta: the physician achievement review. CMAJ 1999;161:52–7.
2. Lockyer JM, Violato C, Fidler H. The assessment of emergency physicians by a regulatory authority. Acad Emerg Med 2006;13:1296–303.
3. Mastenbroek NJ, van Beukelen P, Demerouti E, et al. Effects of a 1 year development programme for recently graduated veterinary professionals on personal and job resources: a combined quantitative and qualitative approach. BMC Vet Res 2015;11:311.
4. Miller A, Archer J. Impact of workplace based assessment on doctors' education and performance: a systematic review. BMJ 2010;341:c5064.
5. Violato C, Lockyer JM, Fidler H. Changes in performance: a 5-year longitudinal study of participants in a multi-source feedback programme. Med Educ 2008; 42:1007–13.
6. Tucker A. Chairing the academic department, leadership among peers. 3rd edition. Phoenix (AZ): Oryx Press; 1993.
7. Buckingham M, Coffman C. First, Break all the Rules : what the World's greatest managers do differently. New York: Simon and Schuster; 1999.
8. Coomer K, Houdmont J. Contribution of work ability and core self-evaluations to worker health. Occup Med (Lond) 2019;69:366–71.
9. Kaplan SH, Griffith JL, Price LL, et al. Improving the reliability of physician performance assessment: identifying the "physician effect" on quality and creating composite measures. Med Care 2009;47:378–87.
10. Hanchak NA, Schlackman N. The measurement of physician performance. Qual Manag Health Care 1995;4:1–12.
11. Kampkötter P. Performance appraisals and job satisfaction. Int J Hum Resource Manag 2017;28:750–74.
12. Epitropaki O, Martin R. From Ideal to Real: A Longitudinal Study of the Role of Implicit Leadership Theories on Leader-Member Exchanges and Employee Outcomes. J Appl Psychol 2005;90:659–76.
13. DiMatteo MR, DiNicola DD. Sources of assessment of physician performance: a study of comparative reliability and patterns of intercorrelation. Med Care 1981; 19:829–42.
14. Dubinsky I, Jennings K, Greengarten M, et al. 360-degree physician performance assessment. Healthc Q 2010;13:71–6.
15. Ramsey PG, Wenrich MD, Carline JD, et al. Use of peer ratings to evaluate physician performance. JAMA 1993;269:1655–60.
16. Kazandjian VA. Power to the people: taking the assessment of physician performance outside the profession. CMAJ 1999;161:44–5.
17. Mozayan C, Manella H, Chimelski E, et al. Patient feedback in the emergency department: A feasibility study of the Resident Communication Assessment Program (ReCAP). J Am Coll Emerg Physicians Open 2020;1:1194–8.
18. Park J-A, Johnson DA, Moon K, et al. The interaction effects of frequency and specificity of feedback on work performance. J Organizational Behav Manag 2019;39:164–78.
19. Le Grand Rogers R, Narvaez Y, Venkatesh AK, et al. Improving emergency physician performance using audit and feedback: a systematic review. Am J Emerg Med 2015;33:1505–14.

Leading and Influencing Culture Change

Christopher A. Adin, DVM, DACVS*

KEYWORDS

- Veterinary • Change management • Leadership • Culture • Barriers

KEY POINTS

- People resist changing behavioral norms, even if the current culture is destructive.
- Leaders must overcome this resistance by providing information to employees, creating a sense of urgency, maintaining an open dialogue, and engaging them in the process.
- Change should be centered on achieving a vision (what can our practice be like) that is understood and shared by all.
- Use positive psychology and identify clear actions that are required to achieve the goal.
- Generate short-term "wins" to provide encouragement.
- Do not stop talking about the change, rewarding good behavior, and removing obstacles until it becomes part of the culture.

INTRODUCTION

Veterinary medicine is changing rapidly as corporate practices; new technologies; low-stress handling; demand for 24-hour care; growth of specialty services; concerns about veterinary well-being; and increasing demands for diversity, equity, and inclusion force practices to evolve or become outmoded. However, human beings have an innate desire to establish and enforce social norms within a group, also known as "culture," even if they become detrimental to both the individual and the group.[1–3] Understanding this phenomenon is essential to achieving strategic change in your practice and is summarized by the famous management consultant, Peter Drucker, in his quote: "Culture eats strategy for breakfast." For this reason, leadership strategies in the last century have followed a 3-step pattern that was proposed by Lewin in 1947: a leader must anticipate and remove resistance to change (unfreeze), seek early wins, and build momentum (manage the change) until the change becomes a behavioral norm in your team (refreeze).[3–5]

Chair and Professor, Department of Small Animal Clinical Sciences, University of Florida, Gainesville, FL, USA
* Corresponding author.
E-mail address: adinc@ufl.edu

Vet Clin Small Anim 51 (2021) 1071–1078
https://doi.org/10.1016/j.cvsm.2021.04.018
0195-5616/21/© 2021 Elsevier Inc. All rights reserved.

INFLUENCING CHANGE

In his book *Influencer, The New Science of Leading Change*, Joseph Grenny and his coauthors argue that organizations are composed of people, and as a result, any change will require a specific change in behavior.[6] In order to be successful, a leader must be skilled in identifying the change in behavior that is required. Most organizations focus on mistakes and how to avoid them, but this negative psychology approach tends to produce little motivation in employees. Modern leaders have learned that you must use positive psychology and look for successes. When someone stands out from the rest and is achieving the outcomes that you want (increased patient safety, good client communication, etc.), find out what it is that they are doing differently than everyone else.[2] This approach is called affinity modeling—looking for "positive deviants" that are uniquely successful in your practice, then figuring out the key behaviors that set them apart.[2,6]

Barriers to Change

Millions of Web sites share the statistic that 70% of change efforts fail. However, critical evaluation of the literature shows that this widely quoted is not based on data but was an "unscientific estimate" that was incorporated into the business management literature because it gave credence to a commonly held belief that change is difficult.[7] In fact, scholars recognize that it is almost impossible to summarize the success rate of change efforts with a single statistic because outcome measures are often insufficient to detect meaningful change. Although experts debate these finer points, all agree that there are common barriers to change and that anticipation of these barriers can help to avoid common mistakes in leading strategic change within a veterinary practice.

Inertia

Newton's first law of physics describes that an object that is stationary tends to remain stationary and resist any change in its current state. Workplace culture follows a similar pattern and must be overcome by a force that will be large enough to overcome the state of inertia. In a business, this energy is supplied by providing evidence and creating a sense of urgency—without this, failure of a change movement is inevitable.[8] You will need to provide your team with data and examples from other practices that will demonstrate the advantages of making your proposed changes, while also providing transparency about the potential risks of making the change. Next, you will need to create a shared vision of what your practice will look like when the new behaviors are incorporated into your culture. Communication about the vision and the change should become part of everything that you do—you must model the change yourself, discuss it in your meetings, advertise it in your newsletters, and call it out when you see someone acting out the change that you are seeking. Every employee from the practice owner to the kennel workers should be able to tell you what the practice vision is and what behaviors are required to get there.

Bad Timing

In his "STARS" model, Michael D. Watkins recognizes that the receptivity of a team to change is largely based on their perceptions of the state of the business or practice.[9] For example, employees in a new practice (a "Start-up"), a practice that is under new ownership (a "Turnover") or one that is experiencing "Accelerated Growth", will generally understand that the situation faced by the business is likely to require change. However, if you are the leader of a practice that has been successful and needs only a gentle "Realignment," or worse, a practice that has "Sustained excellence," it will be much more difficult to create a sense of urgency and explain the need to change so that your practice can reach the next level. Recognizing where your practice is on this scale is essential to understanding and predicting the environment for instituting change. Logically, stable, well-functioning organizations typically require smaller, incremental changes to avoid disruption of a culture that is currently working well. Other investigators have noted that a shock or major disruption is required to create receptivity to change and that without this, significant resistance should be expected.[10]

Nay-Sayers

Leaders typically spend most of their time and effort communicating with "nay-sayers"—those problematic employees who are chronically unhappy and are resistant to change. Any leader will admit that this approach rarely leads to successful change; although the nay-sayers are attention seeking, they are not generally seen as opinion leaders by a team and most will never change. To achieve successful strategic change, you must identify key opinion leaders who are open to change and then join with them to focus on influencing the larger group of employees who are "undecided" but open to change. Unfortunately, the "nay-sayers" will need to either join in or miss the boat.

WHAT SHOULD YOU CHANGE?

It is self-evident that the impact of any change in your practice will depend completely on your ability to select the correct thing to change. We all make thousands of decisions each day, but in their book *Influencer: The New Science of Leading Change*, Grenny and his coauthors assert that there are certain "crucial moments" in the day of an employee that will have a disproportionate effect on the outcomes for the practice. The key for a leader is to identify these crucial moments and to determine what is the behavior or action that is required to achieve the best outcome. The behaviors are typically obvious (described as "Duh" ideas) but need to be identified and called out. As an example from veterinary practice, many small-animal hospitals have 2 different concentrations of enrofloxacin: 22.7 mg/mL is labeled for use in dogs and 100 mg/mL is labeled for use in cattle but is often used topically as a therapy in small animals with skin or ear conditions. If you have had patients receive overdoses of intravenous enrofloxacin due to selection of the wrong bottle when drawing up the injection, what is the vital behavior that can prevent that medical error? Technicians and doctors must develop a habit of reading the concentration and name of the drug on the vial as they are drawing up the drug. It should be a norm—something that will prevent medication errors across all drugs in the hospital but needs to be called out, reinforced, and rewarded in order to make it part of the culture. If you do not see someone doing it, say something! That is how change occurs.

At times, it can be difficult to identify the vital behavior that will lead to the change that is needed in your practice. Searching the literature for evidence-based strategies is a proven approach; however, veterinary practices vary widely and you may need to use different strategies to identify a strategy that will work within your own environment. Solutions that work within your own practice are best identified by looking for "positive deviants"—people who are successful at achieving good outcomes *within your own workplace*. After identifying these personnel, find out how their approach is different from their peers: when they face those "crucial moments" during the day, what action sets them apart from others? Through this method of analysis, you will identify solutions that have already been tested and proved to be effective, despite the challenges within your unique practice environment.

In some cases, a leader will identify that a negative aspect of the culture is what needs to change. Grenny and his coauthors use a story about Delancey Street Foundation, an organization that uses ex-convicts and has shown incredible success by creating vital behaviors that reverse the negative cultural norms that these workers have developed as protective mechanisms. For example, the "care only about yourself" mentality is countered by the vital behavior "take responsibility for someone else's success," with each person being responsible for mentoring another worker. "Don't be a rat" is countered with "everyone confronts everyone else about every single violation." Through these vital behaviors, the leaders create what the authors call "culture busters": actions that reverse the cultural norms, converting destructive behaviors into vital behaviors that lead to organizational success.

THE PROCESS OF CHANGE MANAGEMENT

Although Lewin's general theory of unfreezing the culture, instituting the change, and refreezing the culture seems to accurately reflect the process of successful change, it lacks the detailed steps that are needed to guide new leaders to achieving consistent success.[5] Kotter's famous article in the *Harvard Business Review* in 1995 presented an 8-step guide for this process, which was updated and fleshed out in his book *Accelerate* in 2014, essentially providing an instruction manual for leaders who are seeking to accomplish organizational change (**Table 1**).[8,11] It is important to note that Kotter has now acknowledged that the 8-step process should not be considered in a linear manner but that there will be overlap and simultaneous activation of numerous steps as your practice works to change behaviors, communicate, and adapt to unforeseen challenges.[11,12]

Unfreezing

Urgency
The process of change involves effort and loss. Before your employees will be open to changing their culture, they must be convinced that it is necessary and, furthermore, that it is urgent. Generally, businesses change to increase profits or to improve efficiency or efficacy. This may sound materialistic, but when a broad view is taken, you can see that all issues will boil down to these points. For example, a toxic work environment causes employee turnover, which is both expensive and inefficient for the practice to deal with over time. A practice leader must gather evidence to support

Table 1	
Lewin's foundational "Changing as Three Steps" model is shown to align with the more prescriptive process proposed in Kotter's 8-step process for institutional change[4,8,11]	
Unfreeze the culture	• Create a sense of urgency • Build a coalition of opinion leaders • Form the strategic vision and initiatives • Enlist a volunteer army
Enact the change	• Enable action by removing barriers • Generate short-term wins to increase credibility • Sustain momentum by rewarding early adopters
Freeze the new culture	• Institutionalize and solidify the change as part of the culture

the rationale for change by studying the market and evaluating practice standards, identifying an opportunity that fits their practice, and then be able to present a compelling story to their staff. In communicating about the opportunity for growth, it is important to convey the potential gains associated with succeeding, as well as the costs of failing to adapt and incorporate the change. Communication should be carried out through all available mechanisms and is not successful until every single person in your practice, from kennel worker to Medical Director, is able to recite the rationale for change.

Build a coalition
Leaders will often attempt to shoulder all of the responsibility for change management single-handedly, out of concern that it would be burdensome to ask others to share the load or worse, they cannot trust others to responsibly and skillfully carry the movement. However, a "top-down" approach is doomed to fail from the outset, lacking the buy-in and diversity of ideas that are gained by involving employees from multiple levels of the practice (techs, receptionists, doctors). In selecting this team, Grenny and others suggest that it is important to choose opinion leaders—people who others look to for leadership among their peers.[6] Opinion leaders can be identified through your own observations, but the author has found it more credible to allow peer groups from each level of the organization to select their representatives by holding an anonymous vote, allowing the "people" to decide who will serve as their voice. This team is integral to the success of your strategic change movement and should be involved in every decision and discussion throughout the remaining process.

Form the strategic vision and initiatives
After identifying an opportunity for improving your practice, the strategic planning process must begin by creating a vision for the future. To generate a vision statement, answer the question "how will the future be different from the past and how will we get there?" Kotter asserts that a vision statement must capture the imagination and passion of the employees in a way that data cannot.[11] To do this, he recommends that the vision statement should be generated by team (not by the leader, alone) and that it should be "communicable, desirable, flexible, feasible, imaginable, simple, and should create a verbal picture of the future".[11] People gain understanding through logic, but they get passionate when vision statements are given a more human and emotional appeal. Furthermore, the coalition must define 2 to 3 specific actions that are essential to achieve that vision, using the question: "How do we achieve this goal?"

Enlist a volunteer army
Once a desirable and motivating vision of the future is described and communicated, a significant portion of the employees at your practice must "buy-in" to this vision and embrace the actions that are described in your strategic plan. Kotter suggests that 50% buy-in must be achieved for adoption of change, but even 15% is enough to build momentum as you begin to leverage your communication strategies, reinforce positive behaviors in early adopters, and work with your opinion leaders to convert others to the cause.[6,8,11]

Enacting the Change

Enable action by removing barriers
What rules, policies, or procedures are standing in the way of the strategic actions that you have chosen to pursue? Influencing change is not only about encouraging good behavior, it is also about creating an environment in your practices that encourages

and supports that behavior. Joseph Grenny identifies 6 sources of influence that can help to encourage change (**Box 1**).[6] Half of these key controllers of change relate to the removal of barriers: ensuring that employees have the skills and knowledge to perform the desired behavior (personal ability), the practice culture provides the help needed to accomplish the behaviors (social ability), and that the facility and infrastructure enables the desired behavior (structural ability). As a leader in your practice, you must consider each of these factors, recognizing that removing obstacles is as important as providing motivation for change.

Generate short-term wins to increase credibility

With any public effort, it is important for participants to see that the team has had an early success and that the outcome supports further effort to solidify that change as part of the normal behavior. In fact, short-term wins are so important that you should not wait for them to happen spontaneously; you should *make sure that they happen* and then purposefully communicate about them with all stakeholders. Kotter suggests that short-term wins are most effective when the actions are clear enough to be repeated by others, clearly tied to the current change initiative, and when they produce results that are broadly beneficial, rather than being personal wins for an individual.[8,11]

Sustain momentum by rewarding early adopters

After a few short-term wins, it is time to fan the fire by revisiting the urgency for change, using your early successes to recruit more supporters and expand the percent of employees with "buy-in." This is a time to provide motivation by rewarding people who are embracing the desired change and by removing any newly discovered barriers as the movement takes hold. Continue making changes to infrastructure to support and enable change. This change may involve new equipment, software, or even reassignment or termination of employees who are obstructing the necessary change in behaviors.

Refreezing

Institutionalize and solidify the change

Many practices are able to generate small efforts toward change and even some short-term wins, but few are able to incorporate the new vital behaviors into their DNA in such a way that it becomes the norm, part of the culture. To achieve this, you will need to draw a clear association between the vital behavior (the change)

Box 1
The 6 influencers of change, adapted from Grenny and coauthors' *Influencer: the New Science of Leading Change*, page 70[6]

- Personal Motivation—does the *employee want to* accomplish the vital behavior needed for change?

- Personal Ability—*can* the employee accomplish the vital behavior that is needed?

- Social Motivation—do *others encourage* the vital behavior?

- Social Ability—do *others provide help*, information, or resources to enable the vital behavior?

- Structural Motivation—does the *workplace reward people* who embrace the vital behavior?

- Structural Ability—do the *facility, infrastructure,* and *technology* encourage the vital behavior?

and the good outcomes that are being achieved. Never forget how you got where you are — it was through motivating people to do the desired behavior and by removing any barriers in your practice that are discouraging the changes you seek.

EFFECT OF PRACTICE TYPE

Large academic or public institutions are known to have hierarchical structures with approaches that are dictated by laws or university policies. Although there are fewer studies documenting the strategies for change in public institutions, evidence does exist that change can be enacted with a modification of the 8-step process described earlier.[13] A key difference that distinguishes public institutions and universities from the approaches used in private practices is that leaders will need to garner support from external political forces in addition to building urgency within the organization.[13] If change within a unit, such as a college of veterinary medicine, or a county animal shelter, is not aligned with existing policies and supported by the overseeing board of trustees or the county commissioner, it is doomed from the outset. This additional burden, along with a reputation for slow change within larger institutions can lead to an overestimation of resistance to change, whereas in fact, many individuals within a public organization may be open to and even yearning for change to occur.[13] Tapping into this base of support is a key method for enacting change in larger organizations, not letting the apparent obstacles prevent a leader from enacting needed reforms. In particular, leaders of veterinary practices must realize that traditional management theory that involves a rigid, hierarchical pattern for decision-making is poorly suited for health care and will lead to frustrated employees and high turnover. Veterinary medicine is complex; unpredictable and unique circumstances are faced by highly independent and intelligent veterinarians every day. A rigid approach to a fluid situation will fail, and it must be replaced by relationship-centered administration where leaders are more likely to ask: "What do *you* think we should do?" instead of saying: "Do this."

SUMMARY

As a surgeon performing a difficult procedure, leaders who hope to enact change in their practice must be prepared before starting out and should have a plan that is broken into discrete steps. Human beings are resistant to change, and attempts to change even the most basic of processes (eg, medical records standards, prescription methods, etc.) will not be adopted without significant effort and follow-through on the path of the leader. Thankfully, change management has been studied and discussed extensively by experienced leaders from many disciplines. Veterinarians who are placed in a leadership role in their practice will be far more likely to succeed in changing the culture when they understand how to influence their personnel, can predict common barriers to change, and when they use the processes described in this chapter.

CLINICS CARE POINTS

- Don't waste time trying to convince "naysayers" (those who oppose everything new), focus instead on winning over the positive opinion leaders in your team- the people that everyone looks up to.
- While change is often readily accepted in a business or team that is floundering, it is difficult to enact meaningful change in an organization that is doing well.

DISCLOSURE

The author has nothing to disclose.

REFERENCES

1. Stanford M. The cultural evolution of human nature. Acta Biotheor 2020;68: 275–85.
2. Suchman A, Sluyter D, Williamson P. Leading change in healthcare, transforming organizations using complexity, positive psychology and relationship centered care. New York, NY: Radcliffe Publishing; 2011.
3. Burnes B. Kurt Lewin and the planned approach to change: a re-appraisal. J Manag Stud 2004;41:977–1002.
4. Hussain ST, Lei S, Akram T, et al. Kurt Lewin's change model: a critical review of the role of leadership and employee involvement in organizational change. J Innovation Knowledge 2018;3:123–7.
5. Lewin K. Frontiers in group dynamics: concept, method and reality in social science; social equilibria and social change. Hum Relations 1947;1:5–41.
6. Joseph G, Kerry P, David M, et al. Influencer: the new science of leading change. Second Edition (Paperback). New York: McGraw-Hill; 2013.
7. Hughes M. Do 70 per cent of all organizational change initiatives really fail? J Change Manag 2011;11:451–64.
8. Kotter J. Leading change: why transformation efforts fail. Harv Bus Rev 1995; 73(2):59–67.
9. Watkins MD. The first 90 days: proven strategies for getting up to speed faster and smarter. Boston, MA: Harvard Business Review Press; 2013.
10. Van de Ven A, Poole M. Explaining development and change in organizations. Acad Manage Rev 1993;20:510–40.
11. Kotter JP. Accelerate! Harv Bus Rev 2012;90:45–58.
12. Kotter International. 8-Steps to accelerate change in your organization. 2018. Available at: https://www.kotterinc.com/wp-content/uploads/2019/2004/2018-Steps-eBook-Kotter-2018.pdf. Accessed February 18, 2021.
13. Fernandez S, Rainey H. Managing organizational change in the public sector. Public Adm Rev 2006;66(2):168–76.

Veterinary Clinical Ethics and Patient Care Dilemmas

Callie Fogle, DVM[a],*, Joanne Intile, DVM, MS[b], Mary Katherine Sheats, DVM, PhD[c]

KEYWORDS

- Ethics/veterinary ethics • Communication • Ethical dilemmas • Patient care

KEY POINTS

- Veterinary ethical dilemmas can be classified into 4 categories: autonomy (of the surrogate decision maker), beneficence, justice, and nonmaleficence.
- A structured approach to ethical decision making includes examination of the facts, identification of associated ethical principles, defining stakeholders, generation of alternatives, careful deliberation of alternatives/pertinent moral considerations, selection of the best alternative, and evaluation of the outcome.
- Ethical dilemmas contribute to stress and burnout among veterinarians and staff.
- Veterinarians can use the 4Es approach to address ethical dilemmas: name it, address it, and then enlist, empathize, educate, and engage with resources, clients, and members of the veterinary health care team, as needed.
- Knowledge of communication models and core communication skills can help veterinarians be intentional in framing conversations around ethical dilemmas.

INTRODUCTION

Veterinarians and veterinary technicians encounter complex decisions daily. Some of these dilemmas can be resolved using communication skills and shared decision making with the animal's owner. However, many of these dilemmas are ethical and have no easy solution. Ethical dilemmas are stressful, in part, because they often involve 2 or more choices in direct conflict with each other. Veterinarians can reduce stress associated with these conflicts through knowledge of ethical principles and a deliberate approach to ethical decision making. However, this deliberate approach to ethical decision making is not covered by the code of ethics provided by many veterinary associations and is infrequently taught by veterinary curricula. Consequently,

a Equine Surgery, Department of Clinical Sciences, North Carolina State University-College of Veterinary Medicine, 1060 William Moore Drive, Raleigh, NC 27607, USA; b Medical Oncology, Department of Clinical Sciences, North Carolina State University, 1060 William Moore Drive, Raleigh, NC 27607, USA; c Equine Primary Care, Department of Clinical Sciences, North Carolina State University, 1060 William Moore Drive, Raleigh, NC 27607, USA
* Corresponding author.
E-mail address: cafogle@ncsu.edu

Vet Clin Small Anim 51 (2021) 1079–1097
https://doi.org/10.1016/j.cvsm.2021.05.003
vetsmall.theclinics.com

many veterinarians feel overwhelmed when confronted with an ethical conflict for which there is no easy answer.

Veterinary medical ethics share similarities with human biomedical ethics. Many of the ethical dilemmas in both human and veterinary medicine arise from the desire for, and ability to perform, technologically advanced diagnostics and therapies.[1] Veterinary ethical theory and principles are extrapolated from human biomedical ethics, primarily because the formal study of human biomedical ethics predates the study of veterinary ethics by decades.[2,3] Despite similarities, there are important ethical challenges unique to veterinary medicine.

Animals now have significant moral value in society. A 2015 Gallup poll revealed 32% of Americans believe animals possess a moral value equivalent to humans. Another 62% of Americans believe animals possess moral value but less than humans, such that animals can still be used for the benefit of humans.[4]

The relative moral value possessed by animals is important to a discussion of the conflict between the interests of humans and those of animals. The way in which people ascribe moral value to animals is determined by a variety of cultural norms, such as supporting trophy hunting or even the act of advocating for pet ownership. Perception of an animal's cognitive abilities, sentience, and "human-ness" also contributes to the perception of its moral value.[5,6] The issue is further complicated by societal practices that clearly ascribe different moral value to certain animal species.[7] For example, in some countries, pigs are slaughtered for food, whereas dogs and cats are kept as companions, even though all 3 species feel pain and are of similar intelligence. Animals' moral value has a bearing on everyday decision making within veterinary practice, and the increasing moral value of animals has driven the demand for advances in veterinary health care.

Humans accept that animals are sentient beings with an essential interest in not experiencing pain.[1,8] Two contrasting ethical theories discuss avoidance of suffering. Utilitarianism holds that the best course of action is one producing the most happiness, or the absence of pain.[8] A utilitarian approach focuses on the consequences of a treatment decision and prioritizes a plan causing the least amount of pain or choosing to euthanize an animal rather than treating a likely incurable disease. In contrast with utilitarianism, the rights theory is less concerned with consequences and more concerned with prioritizing the rights of the living being.[9] Advocates of animal rights theory argue that rights are conferred on the basis of capacity for thought and reason, and the ability to feel pain. Rights theory argues that an animal's ability to feel pain is no less than a human's and their rights to avoid such pain are equal.[10,11] As part of the responsibilities of owning an animal, humans consider themselves ethically bound to prevent or minimize discernible suffering in their animals. Laws prohibiting animal cruelty and neglect and governing humane care and slaughter for food animal species are intended to prevent or minimize pain and suffering in animals. In veterinary practice, individuals differ in their judgment of what constitutes animal suffering, what is a satisfactory response to treatment, and what amount of time an animal should be allowed to live with discomfort or chronic illness.

In the United States, animals are the chattels of their owners. Chattel is a general term referring to the owning of tangible moveable personal property, including animals.[12] As chattels, animals do not possess legal rights. Owners are generally free to do what they wish with their animals, provided there is a reasonable effort to prevent or minimize suffering during the animal's life. In practice, what is considered socially tolerable for animals to endure at the hands of their owners differs among individuals, cultures, animal species (cats, dogs, horses, farm animals, and food animals), and even veterinarians.

Another important difference between human medicine and veterinary medicine is the ability to perform euthanasia. Euthanasia is intended to limit animal suffering and/or humanely provide meat for consumption. Most instances of euthanasia are in these categories, but not always. Convenience euthanasia, defined as euthanasia requested for reasons unrelated to ending suffering, causes significant stress to veterinary professionals.[13–16] Survey data document moral stress experienced by veterinarians asked to perform euthanasia on an animal for reasons not agreed on or based on opinions not shared by the veterinarian.[1,10,13,17–19]

Veterinary medical ethics also differs from human medical ethics because veterinary professionals must consider the interests of the owner, who acts as a surrogate decision maker for the animal. Ideally, the interests of the owner align with the best interests of the animal, but this is not always true. For companion animal owners in particular, the emotional attachment, cultural or religious beliefs around euthanasia, and/or financial constraints can supersede the best option for the animal. For example, veterinarians frequently encounter ethical conflict when an owner cannot afford to treat a beloved companion but does not consent to euthanasia, resulting in the animal experiencing unnecessary pain and suffering.

The ethical responsibilities of veterinarians include supporting the needs of the animal, the needs of the owner, and the needs of society.[20] In addition, veterinarians balance their own financial needs, as well as those of their practices. Further, the public is generally unaware that the financial well-being of the veterinary practice is routinely superseded by the needs of the animal and the owner. Veterinarians experience significant moral stress when owners express concern that the veterinarian made decisions in their animal's care purely in an effort to increase their own financial profit.[21] Veterinarians frequently encounter emotionally charged statements in financial discussions (eg, "I thought you loved taking care of animals") when the owner is presented with a larger-than-expected financial estimate for care of an animal.

CLINICAL APPLICATION OF VETERINARY MEDICAL ETHICS

Four ethical principles, modified from those used in human medicine (**Table 1**),[10,22] can be used to frame and discuss most ethical issues veterinarians face. These 4 terms form the basis of principlism, the theory of ethics most commonly used by human medical ethics committees.[1] Although there are other applicable ethical theories,[3,10] the remainder of this article explains, and shows the application of, the 4 components of principlism.

- Autonomy: acknowledging the client or surrogate decision maker's right to make choices and take actions based on personal beliefs and values
  - In cases where client health and well-being are concerned, use of concrete client behaviors, client capacity for consent, client capacity to understand the illness/treatment, and client ability to adhere to a potential plan is important
- Beneficence: offering and providing care plausibly helping the patient achieve a reasonable goal, avoiding undertreatment or overtreatment, and defining reasonable outcomes
- Justice: ensuring fairness in distribution of resources, including clinician and staff time
- Nonmaleficence: first, do no harm; weighing the risks of treatment, the patient's experience during treatment, and the expectation of quality of life after treatment

A systematic approach to an ethical dilemma in clinical veterinary practice can be applied, using a series of standard questions modeled from those developed by the

Table 1
Veterinary interpretations of principlism

Principle	Veterinary Interpretation	Example
Autonomy	Respect and support the client. Acknowledge the client/animal owner's right to make choices and take actions based on personal beliefs and values	Autonomy holds that a veterinarian should support a client who chooses to euthanize a sick animal rather than pursuing a straightforward effective treatment option that puts a significant financial burden on the client
Beneficence	Actions guided by compassion. Offer and provide care to plausibly help the patient achieve a reasonable goal, avoiding undertreatment or overtreatment, defining reasonable outcomes	Beneficence holds that a veterinarian should provide a client with detailed information on a reasonable outcome for an animal with chronic heart failure and offer palliative treatment options that have a good chance of achieving that outcome
Justice	Provide care fairly and equally. Fairly distribute resources, including clinician and staff time	Justice holds that a veterinarian should provide equal time and resources to a client who is easy-going and friendly, and to a client who is intense and demanding. Imagine a veterinarian has 2 clients with animals being treated for the same condition; 1 is mild mannered and easy-going, the other is anxious, overly concerned, and requests multiple updates daily. Justice holds that the veterinarian should provide equal time to both of these clients
Nonmaleficence	First, do no harm. Avoid inaction that results in harm. Weigh the risks of treatment, the patient's experience during treatment, and expectation of quality of life after treatment	Nonmaleficence holds that a veterinarian should not offer continued supportive care as a viable option to an owner whose animal is definitively diagnosed with a solely surgical or inoperable disease

From Beauchamp TL., Childress JF et al. Principles of Biomedical Ethics. Oxford University Press; 2001; with permission.

Clinical Ethics Committee recently formed at North Carolina State University College of Veterinary Medicine (Appendix 1).

- What is the relevant history? Use supportive evidence and facts within the information gathering phase to ensure future decisions made are based on objective data.
- What are the ethical concerns? Use the 4 ethical principles (autonomy of the caregiver, beneficence, justice, and nonmaleficence) to define the main issues. Are there multiple concerns, and are they in conflict with each other?
- Who are the stakeholders? The group may include veterinarians, technicians and other support staff, and the client or a surrogate decision maker.

- What, if anything, is off the table? What will not be offered, no matter the situation?
- What other guidance is needed? Are there legal or administrative questions?
- How might the stakeholders move forward? What alternatives can be considered?
  - Moral imagination, or creativity in identifying ethical options, is critical for generating alternatives to consider.[23]
  - Choices must be weighed based on consequences for all stakeholders, duties, principles, and implications for personal integrity and character. Often, veterinarians are faced with selecting the least bad of several not good choices.
- Once a choice has been made, reflecting on the outcome can be useful to help stakeholders feel empowered, recognize the imperfection of the process, and learn from experiences over time.

Working through an ethical dilemma in practice requires a transparent process highlighting conflicting principles, recognizing the value and contribution of each ethical interest, engaging all stakeholders, and balancing conflicting principles in the difficult decision.

COMMUNICATION STRATEGIES FOR ETHICAL DILEMMAS

Competence in core communication skills and understanding of patient care models are essential aspects of negotiating ethical dilemmas in veterinary practice. Communication skills can be divided into 3 broad categories: content skills, process skills, and perceptual skills.[24,25] Content skills address the information the veterinarian shares with the client through questions, conversation, sharing of resources, and so forth. Process skills address the way the information is shared, including verbal, nonverbal, and written communication. Perceptual skills address both reasoning and relationship skills, such as cultural awareness, self-awareness, attitudes, and biases. Although these categories make these skills seem separate, they are clearly interrelated because the choices veterinarians make about when, how, and what information to share with their clients should be informed by their perceptual skills.

Taken from human medicine, 4 models for clinician-patient communication provide useful context for the discussion of ethical dilemmas in veterinary medicine: paternalistic, informative, interpretive, and deliberative.[26] In the paternalistic (guardian) model, which is perhaps the most familiar, clinicians use their medical knowledge to decide what is in the best interest of the patient, often soliciting little to none of the patient's perspective. In the informative (consumer) model, the clinician provides all available facts related to the medical condition and leaves it to the patient to choose a course of treatment. In the interpretive (counselor) model, the clinician engages the patient in a discussion regarding the patient's goals and values, gives the patient the facts regarding the diagnosis, and helps the patient select the treatment aligning with the patient's values. In the deliberative (friend) model, the clinician also engages the patient in a discussion of health-related values, offering perspectives the patient might not have considered, and advocates for the patient care based on the worthiness of the outcomes.

Charles and colleagues[27] (1999) combined the interpretive and deliberative models into a single collaborator model. Here, the clinician educates the patient regarding the diagnosis, seeks confirmation of the patient's understanding, solicits patient input regarding treatment priorities and goals, shares professional opinions regarding optimal treatment, and engages the patient in shared decision making regarding care. This collaborator role is evident in relationship-centered care, which has emerged as the preferred model of veterinarian-client communication.[28,29] Preference for this model comes from evidence that relationship-centered care improves satisfaction for both clients and clinicians, improves patient outcomes, and results in fewer malpractice claims.[30–32]

Veterinary education literature identifies communication as a clinical competence consisting of 4 core communication skills: nonverbal communication, open-ended questions, reflective listening, and empathy statements.[28] Nonverbal communication includes body language (eg, facial expressions, body posture, and touch), paralanguage (eg, volume, tone, and speed of speech), spatial relationships (eg, whether individuals are standing or sitting, distance, and barriers), and involuntary autonomic responses conveying underlying emotions (eg, tearing, flushing, and pupil size). Open-ended questions are those requiring more than 1-word or 2-word answers and invite the client to share without narrowing the focus of their response. Reflective listening is a technique used to clarify or confirm the client's meaning and/or emotions by repeating what was said with different words and phrases. This technique, along with open-ended questions, allows veterinarians to not only show interest in the client, but also to ensure that they understand the client's perspective. Empathy is the internal act of putting oneself in someone else's position and imagining what they are feeling. Empathy statements allow the veterinarian to recognize another person's experience in a supportive and caring way.

The 4E model for veterinarian-client communication (Cornell and Kopcha[29]), adopted from Keller and Carrol[33] (1994), is particularly helpful because it combines methods of communication with the medical goals for the client/patient in order to deliver relationship-centered care (**Fig. 1**). In this model, Cornell and Kopcha[29] describe engagement as the first step in the client interview. At this stage, the veterinarian acknowledges the value of the information the client provides regarding the animal and assures the client that the client's perspective has value for the shared decision-making process. Next is empathy. In order to be empathetic, the veterinarian must have a sincere interest in the client's perspective, endeavor to see the situation through the client's lens, and express this understanding in a caring and supportive way. Cornell and Kopcha[29] describe the education portion of the client interview as the stage at which the veterinarian presents facts and opinions regarding the patient's medical condition, as well as diagnostic and treatment options. Checking in on the client's level of understanding and soliciting the client's perspectives, questions, concerns, and priorities is an essential part of educating the client. In the enlistment stage, the veterinarian, having already shared educational information with the client, now encourages the client's informed decision making and commitment to adhere to a course of treatment.

Although Cornell and Kopcha[29] use this model as a stepwise approach from beginning to end of the client-patient encounter, it could also be applied as an approach to ethical dilemmas, which are often well after the initial client meeting. Instead of using the adage "Find it, fix it" to describe the medical problem, it could be the conscious process of naming it, as it pertains to identifying 1 or more of the 4 ethical principles, and addressing it by choosing an appropriate course of action. In a similar manner, the 4E's (engage, empathize, educate, and enlist) could be adapted as action items. Engagement pertains not only to the veterinarian-client relationship but also to other resources the veterinarian can call on to address the dilemma, including colleagues, staff, expert resources, and support structures. Empathy can be directed not only toward the client but also to members of the veterinary care team who might be affected by the ethical dilemma. Education includes not only information that veterinarians share with the clients regarding ethical dilemmas but also education the veterinarians

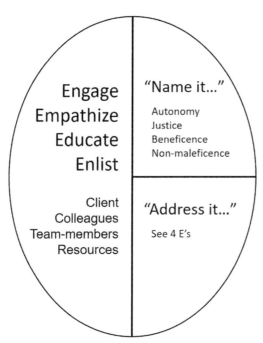

Fig. 1. The 4E model as an approach to veterinary ethical dilemmas. *Adapted from* Cornell KK, Kopcha M. Client-veterinarian communication: skills for client centered dialogue and shared decision making. Vet Clin North Am Small Anim Pract 2007;37(1):37–47; abstract vii. doi: 10.1016/j.cvsm.2006.10.005; with permission.

seeks for themselves, or share with members of the veterinary care team. Enlist describes the process of finding ways to move forward and make decisions regarding ethical dilemmas. The actions and resolutions taken when enlisting the client may be different from those taken when enlisting the veterinary care team, because reflection and a culture of engagement are often an iterative process in veterinary practice.

WHY ARE SKILLS FOR ADDRESSING ETHICAL DILEMMAS IN PRACTICE IMPORTANT?

Ethical dilemmas cause significant stress for veterinarians, veterinary technicians, and/or support staff. A US study showed that 52% of veterinarians identify ethical dilemmas as the leading cause, or one of many equal causes, of work-related stress.[34] Common dilemmas include experiencing unfulfilled moral obligations, conflicting interests of the patient and owner, or competing financial responsibilities of the practice. Veterinary professionals balance complicated ethical questions relating to professional obligations to patients, caretakers, veterinary colleagues, and society. For many veterinary professionals, navigating these conflicts results in intense moral distress, where they know the correct thing to do but feel powerless to do so. Research in human medicine shows moral distress has measurable negative impacts on patient safety, mental health, and professional quality of life, including fostering compassion fatigue.[35,36] Similar associations may exist in veterinary medicine.[37,38] Reducing stakeholders' stress around ethical decision making begins with ensuring all persons feel a strong commitment to their roles in the process and feel supported by the veterinary practice's commitment to ethical standards.[39]

The lack of clearly defined rules of how to approach ethical dilemmas in veterinary medicine further contributes to negative impact on individual well-being. The American Veterinary Medical Association's (AVMA) Principles of Veterinary Medical Ethics states that "the choice of treatments or animal care shall not be influenced by considerations other than the welfare of the patient, the needs of the client, and the safety of the public."[40] This vague statement lacks guidelines necessary for framing the decision-making process for dilemmas encompassing multiple stakeholder's needs. Unsurprisingly, in a survey of methods used to address ethical dilemmas, US veterinarians reported "gut instinct based on their personal value system" as most common, whereas "guidance from written policies of state or national veterinary organizations" and "consideration of varied ethical theories" were used least often.[34] A more helpful strategy is provided by the UK code of conduct acknowledging that, when conflicts in obligations arise, veterinarians are required to rank animal health and welfare as their first concern.[41] Despite stronger verbiage, veterinarians must still interpret what constitutes the act of prioritizing the needs of the animal over the caretaker or public.

A lack of systematic approach to dilemmas is most pronounced in scenarios where the veterinarian faces competing responsibilities to the animal caretaker and the animal and has no obvious way to prioritize one over the other. Hernandez and colleagues[42] note that, "in reality, many ethical dilemmas are 'solved' by prioritizing the interests of the client over the interests of the animal." This approach clearly avoids formulating a decision based on ethical or moral principles, but instead bases it on maintaining a secure relationship with pet owners or caretakers.

Despite the frequency at which veterinarians encounter ethical dilemmas, busy practitioners lack the time and resources to educate themselves on approaches to ethical situations. Although formal teaching of veterinary ethics is mandated by some teaching programs (eg, the AVMA), there is no established curriculum to accomplish this goal. Although there are few studies on veterinary ethics education, evidence shows that experienced veterinarians recognize the importance of (1) increasing student's exposure to realistic cases challenging ethical values, and (2) exposing students to a variety of owner opinions related to ethical scenarios to increase their awareness of diverse values and opinions.[43] Veterinarians also acknowledge the value of, and rely heavily on, their peers as a support network. The need for ethical support and opportunity for individuals to gain insight from others is worth further study in veterinary medicine. A potential model for such action can be found in the mentoring program created by the Australian Veterinary Association, where new graduates have the chance to discuss ethical dilemmas with more experienced colleagues.[44]

CASE EXAMPLES
Case 1

When the owner's interests are in conflict with the animal's interests
Dr Fields is an ambulatory large animal veterinarian in a mixed animal practice. He evaluates a juvenile goat who was rescued 6 months ago from a hoarding situation. He previously diagnosed the goat with malnutrition and severe osteopenia as well as a pathologic left pelvic limb fracture occurring around the time of rescue. The rescue operation was able to obtain funding, and the owner, Ms Boswell, elected to have the left pelvic limb amputated at a nearby referral hospital. The goat did well for a few months, but is now recumbent, with an obvious instability of the right pelvic limb. Dr Fields suspects the goat's unresolved osteopenia contributed to a second pathologic fracture. He discusses his findings with Ms Boswell, who states she would like an emergency referral for a second pelvic limb amputation and fitting for a cart,

before any discussion of treatment options. Dr Fields has concerns about the animal's quality of life, but Ms Boswell is unwilling to listen to those concerns. Dr Fields calls the surgeon in the referral practice and discusses his ethical concerns about offering a second pelvic limb amputation. Dr Fields explains he likely would not have offered referral for a second amputation, because a bilateral amputation in a small ruminant is not common, he does not know whether the goat would tolerate a cart, and he has ongoing concerns about the animal's unresolved osteopenia and risk of additional fractures. The surgeon understands Dr Fields' concerns and is also reluctant to offer a second amputation. The surgeon is unsure whether the practice allows him to refuse to perform a procedure he is technically capable of performing. He discusses this with the practice owner after the phone call ends. Ms Boswell is extremely unhappy when she hears the referral practice may not offer the procedure she wants. She feels Dr Fields has talked the surgeon out of offering this procedure for her goat and expresses a desire to find another nearby referral practice to perform the procedure. Dr Fields persuades Ms Boswell to wait for the surgeon's callback before making any decisions. He stabilizes the goat's leg before leaving the rescue. Later, the surgeon calls Dr Fields to let him know he will not offer a second pelvic limb amputation for the goat, based on the concerns he had expressed. He suggests a conference call to discuss this with Ms Boswell. Together, they discuss all possible options for treatment and the concerns of bilateral pelvic limb amputation in a juvenile goat, in the face of unresolved osteopenia. Dr Fields restates his concerns for the possibility of chronic bloat, intolerance of a cart, and additional limb fractures, and those concerns are emphasized by the surgeon. Ms Boswell is extremely unhappy; she does not want to euthanize such a young animal, but she does finally hear and appreciate their concerns for the animal's quality of life. She decides not to find a second referral hospital willing to perform the procedure, but instead elects to have the goat humanely euthanized at the farm.

Commentary

This case exemplifies a common ethical dilemma veterinarians face: a conflict between the owner's desires for the animal and the veterinarian's perception of the animal's quality of life and what might be in the animal's best interest. At the root of the conflict are the disparate viewpoints: the owner's desire for the animal to have surgery and continue to live, and the veterinarian's belief that subjecting the goat to surgery is likely to result in further suffering. In addition, the owner has a legal right to treat the goat as she wishes, provided suffering is prevented or at least minimized.

Beneficence

Dr Fields has concerns about the animal's quality of life after a bilateral pelvic limb amputation, and whether the procedure will help the goat. There are several unknowns here he must weigh, concerning expectations of the goat's future quality of life. Will the goat tolerate a bilateral pelvic limb amputation? Will it be able to eructate as all ruminant animals must do, or will it develop chronic bloat? Will it tolerate living in a cart? The presence of unresolved osteopenia provides another layer of complexity for Dr Fields. Will the goat simply fracture another limb after the bilateral pelvic limb amputation? These concerns are paramount for Dr Fields.

Autonomy

The goat is legally Ms Boswell's personal property, and she wants the second pelvic limb amputated on the goat. She believes what she is requesting is in the goat's best interest.

Often, in difficult decisions with unrecognized ethical conflicts, veterinarians may decide to prioritize the owner's wishes over their perceptions of the animal's best interest. In this case, Dr Fields was eventually able to communicate his ethical concerns to Ms Boswell, so he could prioritize the animal's quality of life. Dr Fields and the surgeon informally worked through components of the ethical framework during their first and second phone calls. They discussed the relevant facts and Dr Fields shared his ethical concerns. They discussed amputation as a matter of what they would not do, but the surgeon realized he needed the support of the practice to be able to do so. Discussion of additional options did not occur here but could have been another useful component of the conversation. The veterinarian and veterinary surgeon worked as a team during the conference call to show their passion for the goat's best interests and discuss their serious concerns for its future quality of life.

Communication strategies and the 4Es

The use of education as a communication strategy was a prominent feature in this case. Ms Boswell may not have known about the concerns of an inability to eructate and what that means for a ruminant's quality of life. She likely did not know how high the goat's risk was for further limb fractures. In the conference call, Dr Fields and the surgeon were able to give her a different perspective by sharing this information. Ms Boswell was initially resistant to discussing concerns for the goat's quality of life, and use of reflective listening and empathy statements might have helped to lower her defensive barriers. During their initial conversation, Dr Fields could have used reflective listening to recognize Ms Boswell's perspective, such as, "I am hearing you would really like to try the surgery and see if he will tolerate a cart; you want to try to save the goat if at all possible." Dr Fields does not have to agree with Ms Boswell, but he does need to establish her trust, and that begins with letting the client know that she is heard. "I hear the frustration in your voice" is another example of reflective listening that would have been appropriate for this case. "I understand how painful this is. I have lost a young animal too," is an empathy statement that Dr Fields could have used to express caring for Ms Boswell's distress. Engaging Ms Boswell in a discussion of the risks and benefits of performing the procedure, once she was ready to listen, and use of shared decision making to help align treatment options with Ms Boswell's values and goals for her rescued goat were critical to this outcome. In reflecting on this case, it is important to recognize that a different outcome may have been chosen, because different owners and veterinarians can have different ethical frameworks than what was depicted here. Ms Boswell could also have elected to take the goat elsewhere for the procedure, but Dr Fields and the surgeon showed a transparent consideration of all the options, and selection of an alternative aligned with their professional moral standards and was supported by their respective practices.

Case 2

When conflict arises because of resource limitations

Dr Sanchez is the owner of a busy 4-doctor small animal practice in the suburbs of a major US city. In May of 2020, her practice was facing a dilemma. The COVID-19 (coronavirus disease 2019) pandemic created a worldwide shortage in personal protective equipment (PPE), including disposable gloves, long-sleeved gowns, goggles, and face shields. Her practice managed to secure supplies lasting through the month, but they had real concerns about supply chains moving forward. Dr Sanchez knew the clinic needed to reevaluate their protocols to conserve their resources. She also knew medical oncology patients receiving chemotherapeutic agents required extensive PPE for each appointment, and she wondered whether the treatments and/or protocols with these patients could or should be altered.

Commentary

This dilemma is multifactorial and involves the interests of multiple stakeholders. Chemotherapeutics have the ability to extend and even save lives for veterinary patients, and, when medically appropriate, most veterinarians consider them as a viable treatment option to present to clients. However, contact with chemotherapeutics has known risks for humans, and proper protocols, containment devices, and PPE are needed to help mitigate those risks and protect veterinarians, veterinary personnel, and clients. In addition, the COVID-19 pandemic created a global health care crisis and, during the height of this crisis, everyone was asked to conserve PPE for frontline health care workers. In this situation, how should Dr Sanchez and her practice balance the medical needs of their patients, the desires of their clients, the safety of veterinarians and veterinary personnel, the limitation in resources, and the societal interests for, and individual interests of, human health care workers?

Justice

The concept of justice as it relates to medical ethics deals with ensuring fairness regarding distribution of resources. In this scenario, the availability of PPE is limited, and veterinarians must weigh the potential consequences to, and interests of, the different stakeholders in order to determine a fair course of action.

As a first step, Dr Sanchez considered the interests of herself and her staff. Although the use of chemotherapeutics in veterinary species is considered by some to be an ethical issue of its own,[45] their use in the treatment of companion animals is increasing.[46] With increasing use of hazardous drugs (HDs) comes increased risk of human exposure. The National Institute for Occupational Safety and Health (NIOSH) classifies handling of cytotoxic drugs as an occupational hazard, and several states, including Washington, California, and North Carolina, mandate that veterinary hospitals comply with NIOSH guidelines regarding HD safety in the workplace.[46,47] Veterinary personnel are at risk of exposure when receiving, storing, preparing, administering, disposing of, and cleaning up waste from patients treated with HDs. Routes of potential exposure include skin contact, skin absorption, inhalation of aerosols or drug particles, ingestion, and needle-stick injuries. The following minimum PPE is recommended when handling HDs: chemotherapy-rated (ASTM International [formerly American Society Testing Materials]) double-gloving, long-sleeved coated impermeable gown with back closure, shoe coverings, hair coverings to maintain sterility (if needed), eye shield/face shield if potential for splashing/aerosolization, and respirator (fitted).[46] In this scenario, Dr Sanchez and her team put a great deal of effort into creating updated policies and procedures regarding the handling and administration of HDs based on available resources[48,49] and consultation with the veterinary oncology service at a nearby referral hospital. They worked hard to train their personnel and even designated a safety officer. Dr Sanchez knew she needed to talk with her team about this dilemma. She was not sure asking her team to stretch the use of PPE was fair to them in terms of their safety, given how little is known about chemotherapy exposure and adverse outcomes in veterinary medicine.[46] She also did not want to undermine the standards of workplace safety they worked so hard to establish. However, she also knew her team cared deeply about their patients and might find it distressing to stop providing treatment. In addition, she considered the option to limit chemotherapy to medications given per os, which would decrease the use of PPE, but this conflicted with her feelings about her professional obligation to provide the highest level of care possible for her patients and clients.

Other stakeholders in this scenario who are affected by Dr Sanchez's dilemma are human health care workers. Dr Sanchez was acutely aware of the COVID-19 crisis and the devastating toll of the pandemic, but she was not sure how to balance the specific interests of her veterinary patients against the general needs of human health care workers. She also knew her feelings might be different from those of her colleagues. She remembered learning in a veterinary ethics course that people differed in their conceptual approaches to balancing the needs of animals against the needs of people. For example, utilitarianism equates animal welfare with human welfare,[8] whereas Kantian philosophy excludes animals as nonautonomous beings and states that human interests always supersede animal interests, even if animal suffering is the result.[50] Although Dr Sanchez did not personally identify with either of these extremes, she was not sure how to justify a decision that was somewhere in the middle.

Communication strategies and the 4Es

In order to address her dilemma, Dr Sanchez decided to engage a veterinary oncologist colleague at a nearby referral hospital. Her colleague reassured her that she was not alone in her dilemma and shared a modified HDs protocol developed at a college of veterinary medicine designed to conserve PPE without overtly compromising the safety of veterinary personnel. Although Dr Sanchez thought the modified protocol was a viable option, she wanted to avoid a paternalistic model of communication with her team, so she decided to have a meeting with her doctors and staff where she presented the dilemma, the ethical concerns it presented, and the list of stakeholders to consider. Once she was done introducing the topics for the meeting, she sat down, using nonverbal communication to signal she did not want to dominate the conversation and intended to listen to what others had to say. She used open-ended questions, such as "What are your thoughts about this situation?" to encourage dialogue. When team members expressed concern regarding safety or changes to patient care options, she used empathy statements such as, "You know, I had the same thought and it upset me too," to show she cared for and identified with their feelings. Dr Sanchez also chose to educate her team, sharing the modified protocol she was given by a colleague. Once they had all of the relevant information, she asked her team to make a decision about how to move forward, enlisting them to find a resolution.

Case 3

When conflict arises, defining what constitutes not doing harm

Dr Davis is a newly graduated small animal veterinarian working in a busy 2-doctor general practice. Her clinic does not have overnight care but routinely sees emergency patients during the day. Patients requiring overnight care are referred to a local 24-hour emergency clinic. Dr Davis notes a new client on her schedule for the day. The patient is a 4-year-old intact female English bulldog scheduled for a pre-surgery examination. The notes for the appointment state: "Exam prior to scheduled cesarean section (c-section) next week." Dr Davis reviews the dog's medical records and finds the client is a breeder referred to her hospital from a local general practice. This appointment is the patient's second scheduled c-section. Her first surgery was approximately 2 years ago, and was done by Dr Williams, the other veterinarian at the clinic, who is also the practice owner. The patient has not been seen at the clinic since the surgery. Dr Davis asks Dr Williams about the appointment, and the owner indicates it is hospital policy to honor such referrals and she would have seen the patient herself, but she will be out of town next week. She shows enthusiasm for Dr Davis to gain further surgical experience, to maintain the collegial relationship with the referring hospital, and states that she is confident Dr Davis will be fine. Dr Davis is appreciative of her praise but feels uncomfortable with this plan. She has only performed 1 c-section before and has limited experience anesthetizing brachycephalic dogs. In veterinary school, she witnessed a bulldog collapse from respiratory distress while being discharged from a routine wellness appointment. That dog was ultimately euthanized because of the owner's inability to financially support prolonged treatment in the intensive care unit. Dr Davis is also uncomfortable with supporting breeding of brachycephalic dogs.

The following day, Dr Davis asks to meet with Dr Williams and explains her concerns. Dr Williams is unhappy about the prospect of losing the referral and angering the clinic that referred the patient. She maintains that working with the breeder does not contribute to negative animal welfare. Dr Williams feels obligated to provide medical care for the patient and stands by her decision to accept such referrals. After a contentious, but conscientious, discussion, Dr Williams accedes to Dr Davis' request to refer the breeder to another facility. However, she asks Dr Davis to contact the referring hospital and the breeder and explain the need for referral elsewhere. Dr Davis is concerned that she disappointed her employer and harmed her future at her clinic but is relieved to avoid performing the surgery and agrees to make the calls.

Commentary

This case show how ethical considerations can be contradictory, even within the context of a single clinical scenario. On one hand, declining to perform surgery places the dam and her offspring at high risk for a poor outcome, possibly death. In contrast, Dr Williams has a valid concern that her inexperience and the hospital's limitations for care will harm this patient and her puppies. The stakeholders, Dr Davis as the associate, Dr Williams as the practice owner, the breeder, the referral hospital, and the dam and puppies, all have diverse interests to consider. This ethical dilemma highlights the importance of a structured, transparent approach that considers the interests of all stakeholders and uses shared decision making, empathy, and education in resolving ethical conflict.

The ethics of dog breeding

One point of view argues that the very act of engaging in breeding dogs is unethical, because every puppy deliberately produced causes the death of a dog in a shelter. In addition, although survival of the species and reproduction are deeply seated instincts for most organisms, pedigree breeding causes significant and avoidable harms to dogs. A more moderate approach considers ethical or responsible breeding appropriate, while criticizing scenarios such as commercial breeding kennels, backyard breeders, and unplanned matings. In the scenario presented earlier, breeding and conception have already occurred. Therefore, the focus must shift from a debate regarding the ethics of planned reproduction to development of an ethical approach to the patient's current status.

Nonmaleficence. In this scenario, Dr Davis is experiencing conflict around the principle of nonmaleficence, avoiding harm through action as well as through inaction or neglect. She clearly desires to do no harm but must balance the possible harm caused by performing the surgery herself with that caused by refusing to perform the surgery. Because many medical treatments inherently create some amount of harm, veterinarians often weigh the degree and likelihood of harm from the therapy with the chances of a successful outcome and expected benefit.

Overall, mortalities of dams and puppies undergoing c-section in the United States and Canada are low and elective c-section reduces risk for neonatal mortality.[51] However, maternal brachycephaly is a risk factor for early puppy survival, and bitches with prior c-section have a higher risk of obstetric complications than the general obstetric population.[51,52] Considering the principle of nonmaleficence, breed-specific risk data allow Dr Davis to justify her actions either way. If she performs the surgery with the goal of preserving both maternal and fetal life, she is avoiding doing harm. If she declines to perform the surgery because she lacks the necessary resources to ensure an optimal outcome, she is also avoiding doing harm. Dr Davis uses creativity in identifying an additional ethical alternative, the option for external referral of the case to an outside facility. Had this choice not been available, Dr Davis would balance the consequences of performing surgery with refusal to perform surgery, prioritizing the least bad alternative after considering the chances of a good outcome and least likelihood of harm.

Communication strategies and the 4Es

Communication toward the practice owner. New graduates identify confidence in their surgical skills and ability to perform surgery as a top shortcoming of their education.[53,54] Lack of experience is highlighted in a 2018 study that showed almost half of graduating veterinary students had never performed an unassisted canine ovariohysterectomy.[55] Inexperienced veterinarians take longer to complete routine procedures, and increasing length of anesthesia is associated with higher perianesthetic complication rates.[56] Dr Davis read these studies and is extremely concerned her lack of experience and lack of 24-hour care at her practice may lead to an anesthetic complication she will not be able to resolve. Dr Davis has used educate as one of the 4Es to address her ethical dilemma, and her research supports her use of nonmaleficence to frame her dilemma and her decision to decline to perform the surgery.

Before her conversation with Dr Williams, Dr Davis is likely to feel anxious. When preparing for a courageous (ie, difficult) conversation, it is useful for veterinarians to gather an awareness of their levels of stress or anxiety. These feelings can cause acting out in the form of defensiveness and scripted responses, but acting out can be avoided by sharing feelings, maintaining physical relaxation, and being empathetic. Dr Davis could empathize with the position Dr Williams is in as her employer with a statement such as, "This is your practice and my choice affects you too. I understand why you are frustrated." They can both manage their nonverbal cues to ensure open communication by nodding, using a calm tone and consistent eye-contact, and maintaining nonthreatening poses (eg, avoiding crossing arms/legs, lack of frequent hand gestures). They can choose to have the conversation in an environment without distraction. When communication around conflict is authentic and relationship based, it can ultimately increase the respect and trust between colleagues.[57]

Communication with the referring hospital. Effective communication is the foundation for any relationship between practitioners sharing case responsibilities. In this scenario, the referring hospital might be upset that Dr Davis has declined to perform the surgery, even though Dr Davis has made her decision based on ethical reasoning. Dr Davis can use reflective listening and open-ended questions to help preserve a working relationship with the referring hospital. If the referring veterinarian expresses frustration or displeasure with Dr Davis' choice, she can use reflective listening to make sure she is appreciating her colleague's perspective. Reflective listening often begins with phrases such as, "Am I correct that your main concern is....?," "What I am hearing is...," and "Tell me if I have this right: you feel as though....." Although human physicians who used reflective listening were less likely to have a history of malpractice claims,[58] only about 50% of small animal appointments include reflective listening,[59] and many veterinarians do not use it routinely. Open-ended questions could also have been used to invite feedback and signal that Dr Davis is interested in maintaining a good working relationship. Open-ended questions for this situation include, "What can I do to avoid putting you in this position in the future?" or "How can I help you find a surgeon and facility that will achieve your goals for this breeder?" Answers to these questions enlist the referring veterinary hospital in developing a plan for the future.

Communication with the client. In this scenario, the communication with the client is perhaps the most complex. Dr Davis' refusal to perform the c-section is likely to upset the client, and potentially even cause distress. In addition, because Dr Davis is opposed to breeding brachycephalic dogs, she may lack genuine empathy for the client's situation. Dr Davis' communication choices may differ depending on whether she chooses to treat this client with the relationship-based communication model or one of the more removed models, such as paternalistic or informative. It may be difficult for Dr Davis to use the relationship-based model when her values are so divergent from those of the client. Nevertheless, should Dr Davis choose the relationship-based model, she could empathize with the client with statements such as, "I know if I were in your position I would be upset, especially because our hospital has done this surgery for your dog before." She could combine empathy with open-ended questions to elicit the client's perspective: "If my dog was referred for surgery and then refused, I would feel confused. Please tell me how I can help you with what comes next." Veterinarians may not be inclined to use relationship-based communication in every situation, but use of the model does not mean veterinarians have to agree with, or even like, their clients' choices. Use of the model simply offers veterinarians the tools to provide their best effort at communication with diverse clients in various circumstances.

SUMMARY

Veterinary ethical dilemmas are common and unavoidable, inflicting stress on all members of the veterinary team. This stress can be reduced by creating a structure for tackling ethical conflicts that promotes identification of an ethical concern and effective communication of the facts, supports diverse interests of the stakeholders, and enhances transparency around the decision-making process. As a first step in the approach, veterinarians can name their ethical dilemma with 1 or more of the following principles: autonomy, beneficence, justice, and nonmaleficence. In order to address their dilemma, veterinarians can use the 4Es model to enlist, educate, empathize, and engage with resources, clients, and members of the veterinary team. Use of nonverbal communication, reflective listening, open-ended questions, and empathy statements are core communication concepts that veterinarians can use to support themselves, the veterinary team, the practice, and the owner. A practice culture that promotes individual and group reflection on the process and the outcome of ethical dilemmas highlights the missteps and creates a supportive environment where all members feel empowered to participate in, and learn from, the experiences.

ACKNOWLEDGMENTS

The authors acknowledge current and previous members of the North Carolina State College of Veterinary Medicine Clinical Ethics Committee: Philip Rosoff, Jeannine

Moga, Rebecca Maher, Bruce Keene, Chris Adin, Heather Hopkinson, Charity Weyh-rauch, Margaret Gruen, and Stephanie Burgess (Callie Fogle and Joanne Intile are current members) for their efforts in furthering the practice of clinical veterinary ethics. The Clinical Ethics Committee is also acknowledged for creation of the Clinical Ethics Committee form used in this article.

DISCLOSURE

The authors have nothing to disclose.

REFERENCES

1. Rosoff PM, Moga J, Keene B, et al. Resolving ethical dilemmas in a tertiary care veterinary specialty hospital: adaptation of the human clinical consultation committee model. Am J Bioeth 2018;18(2):41–53.
2. Jonsen AR. The birth of bioethics. Hastings Cent Rep 1993;23(6):1.
3. Rollin BE. An introduction to veterinary medical ethics : theory and cases. Ames (IA): Wiley-Blackwell; 2006.
4. Gallup. In U.S., More Say Animals Should Have Same Rights as People. 2015. Available at: https://news.gallup.com/poll/183275/say-animals-rights-people.aspx. Accessed February 13, 2021.
5. Mullan S, Quain A, Wensley S. Veterinary ethics : navigating Tough cases. Sheffield (UK): 5m Publishing; 2017.
6. Adin CA, Moga JL, Keene BW, et al. Clinical ethics consultation in a tertiary care veterinary teaching hospital. J Am Vet Med Assoc 2019;254(1):52–60.
7. Coeckelbergh M, Gunkel DJ. Facing animals: a relational, other-oriented approach to moral standing. J Agric Environ Ethics 2014;27(5):715–33.
8. Bentham J, Burns JH, Hart HLA. An Introduction to the Principles of Morals and Legislation. Oxford: Oxford University Press; 1996. p. 11–34.
9. Francione G. Reflections on "Animals, Property, and the Law" and "Rain without Thunder". Anim L Policy 2007;70(1):9–57.
10. Sandøe P, Corr S, Palmer C. Companion animal ethics. New York: John Wiley & Sons, Inc; 2015.
11. Cochrane A. Ownership and Justice for Animals. Utilitas 2009;21(4):424–42.
12. Definition of CHATTEL. Available at: https://www.merriam-webster.com/dictionary/chattel. Accessed February 13, 2021.
13. Cholbi M. The Euthanasia of Companion Animals. In: Overall C, editor. Pets and people: the ethics of companion animals. New York: Oxford University Press; 2017. p. 1–16.
14. O'Connor E. Sources of work stress in veterinary practice in the UK. Vet Rec 2019;184(19):588.
15. Scotney RL, McLaughlin D, Keates HL. A systematic review of the effects of euthanasia and occupational stress in personnel working with animals in animal shelters, veterinary clinics, and biomedical research facilities. J Am Vet Med Assoc 2015;247(10):1121–30.
16. Correction. A systematic review of the effects of euthanasia and occupational stress in personnel working with animals in animal shelters, veterinary clinics, and biomedical research facilities. J Am Vet Med Assoc 2016;248(3):281.
17. Hart LA, Hart BL, Mader B. Humane euthanasia and companion animal death: caring for the animal, the client, and the veterinarian. J Am Vet Med Assoc 1990;197(10):1292–9.

18. Yeates JW, Main DCJ. Veterinary opinions on refusing euthanasia: justifications and philosophical frameworks. Vet Rec 2011;168(10):263.

19. Yeates JW, Main DCJ. The ethics of influencing clients. J Am Vet Med Assoc 2010;237(3):263–7.

20. Bones VC, Yeates JW. The emergence of veterinary oaths: social, historical, and ethical considerations. J An Ethics 2012;2(1):20–42.

21. Coe JB, Adams CL, Bonnett BN. A focus group study of veterinarians' and pet owners' perceptions of the monetary aspects of veterinary care. J Am Vet Med Assoc 2007;231(10):1510–8.

22. Beauchamp TL, Childress JF, et al. Principles of biomedical ethics. New York: Oxford University Press; 2001.

23. Hartman L, DesJardins J, MacDonald C. Business ethics: decision making for personal integrity & social responsibility. New York: McGraw-Hill; 2020.

24. Chadderdon LM, King LJ, Lloyd JW. The skills, knowledge, aptitudes, and attitudes of successful veterinarians: a summary of presentations to the NCVEI subgroup (Brook Lodge, Augusta, Michigan, December 4-6, 2000). J Vet Med Educ 2001;28(1):28–30.

25. Silverman J, Kurtz S, Draper J. Skills for communicating with patients. Arbingdon (UK): Radcliffe Medical Press; 2005.

26. Emanuel EJ, Emanuel LL. Four models of the physician-patient relationship. JAMA 1992;267(16):2221–6.

27. Charles C, Gafni A, Whelan T. Decision-making in the physician-patient encounter: revisiting the shared treatment decision-making model. Soc Sci Med 1999;49(5):651–61.

28. Shaw JR. Four core communication skills of highly effective practitioners. Vet Clin North Am Small Anim Pract 2006;36(2):385–96, vii.

29. Cornell KK, Kopcha M. Client-veterinarian communication: skills for client centered dialogue and shared decision making. Vet Clin North Am Small Anim Pract 2007;37(1):37–47 [abstract vii].

30. Hall JA, Dornan MC. Meta-analysis of satisfaction with medical care: description of research domain and analysis of overall satisfaction levels. Soc Sci Med 1988;27(6):637–44.

31. Stewart MA. Effective physician-patient communication and health outcomes: a review. CMAJ 1995;152(9):1423–33.

32. Levinson W. Physician-patient communication. A key to malpractice prevention. JAMA 1994;272(20):1619–20.

33. Keller VF, Carroll JG. A new model for physician-patient communication. Patient Educ Couns 1994;23(2):131–40.

34. Kipperman B, Morris P, Rollin B. Ethical dilemmas encountered by small animal veterinarians: characterisation, responses, consequences and beliefs regarding euthanasia. Vet Rec 2018;182(19):548.

35. Christodoulou-Fella M, Middleton N, Papathanassoglou EDE, et al. Exploration of the association between nurses' moral distress and secondary traumatic stress syndrome: implications for patient safety in mental health services. Biomed Res Int 2017;2017:1908712.

36. Austin CL, Saylor R, Finley PJ. Moral distress in physicians and nurses: Impact on professional quality of life and turnover. Psychol Trauma 2017;9(4):399–406.

37. Roff S. Only connect: a web-based approach to supporting student learning in the philosophy of social science. Discourse Learn Teach Philos Relig Stud 2009;8(2):197–207.

38. Kahler SC. Moral stress the top trigger in veterinarians' compassion fatigue: veterinary social worker suggests redefining veterinarians' ethical responsibility. J Am Vet Med Assoc 2015;246(1):16–8.
39. Fisher CB, True G, Alexander L, et al. Moral stress, moral practice, and ethical climate in community-based drug-use research: views from the front line. AJOB Prim Res 2013;4(3):27–38.
40. Principles of Veterinary Medical Ethics of the AVMA. Available at: https://www-avma-org.prox.lib.ncsu.edu/resources-tools/avma-policies/principles-veterinary-medical-ethics-avma. Accessed February 13, 2021.
41. Royal College of Veterinary Surgeons. Code of Professional Conduct for Veterinary Surgeons. Available at: https://www.rcvs.org.uk/setting-standards/advice-and-guidance/code-of-professional-conduct-for-veterinary-surgeons/pdf/. Accessed February 13, 2021.
42. Hernandez E, Fawcett A, Brouwer E, et al. Speaking up: veterinary ethical responsibilities and animal welfare issues in everyday practice. Animals (Basel) 2018;8(1):15.
43. Richards L, Coghlan S, Delany C. "I had no idea that other people in the world thought differently to me": ethical challenges in small animal veterinary practice and implications for ethics support and education. J Vet Med Educ 2020;47(6):728–36.
44. Australian Veterinary Association. Graduate Mentoring Program. Available at: https://www.ava.com.au/about-us/programs-awards/graduate-mentoring-program/. Accessed February 13, 2021.
45. Stephens T. The Use of Chemotherapy to Prolong the Life of Dogs Suffering from Cancer: The Ethical Dilemma. Animals (Basel) 2019;9(7):441.
46. Smith AN, Klahn S, Phillips B, et al. ACVIM small animal consensus statement on safe use of cytotoxic chemotherapeutics in veterinary practice. J Vet Intern Med 2018;32(3):904–13.
47. National Institute for Occupational Safety and Health. Safe Handling of Hazardous Drugs for Veterinary Healthcare Workers. 2010;2021.
48. Biller B, Berg J, Garrett L, et al. 2016 AAHA Oncology Guidelines for Dogs and Cats. J Am Anim Hosp Assoc 2016;52(4):181–204.
49. Steffy-Morgan JD. Chemotherapy: Chemotherapy Administration. In: Henry CJ, Higginbotham ML, editors. Cancer Management in Small Animal practice; 2010. Maryland Heights, MO: Saunders Elsevier. 114-118.
50. Alexander B, Elizabeth MP. Kant's treatment of animals. Philosophy 1974;49(190):83–375.
51. Moon PF, Erb HN, Ludders JW, et al. Perioperative management and mortality rates of dogs undergoing cesarean section in the United States and Canada. J Am Vet Med Assoc 1998;213(3):365–9.
52. DeCramer KGM. 2017. Preparturient caesarean section in the bitch: justification, timing, execution, and outcome evaluation. Doctoral dissertation. University of Pretoria, Pretoria, South Africa. Corpus ID: 116044882.
53. Cary JA, Farnsworth CH, Gay J, et al. Stakeholder expectations regarding the ability of new veterinary graduates to perform various diagnostic and surgical procedures. J Am Vet Med Assoc 2017;251(2):172–84.
54. Routly JE, Taylor IR, Turner R, et al. Support needs of veterinary surgeons during the first few years of practice: perceptions of recent graduates and senior partners. Vet Rec 2002;150(6):167–71.
55. Gates MC, Odom TF, Sawicki RK. Experience and confidence of final year veterinary students in performing desexing surgeries. N Z Vet J 2018;66(4):210–5.

56. Gruenheid M, Aarnes TK, McLoughlin MA, et al. Risk of anesthesia-related complications in brachycephalic dogs. J Am Vet Med Assoc 2018;253(3):301–6.
57. Kurtz S. Teaching and learning communication in veterinary medicine. J Vet Med Educ 2006;33(1):11–9.
58. Levinson W, Roter DL, Mullooly JP, et al. Physician-patient communication. The relationship with malpractice claims among primary care physicians and surgeons. JAMA 1997;277(7):553–9.
59. Shaw JR, Adams CL, Bonnett BN. What can veterinarians learn from studies of physician-patient communication about veterinarian-client-patient communication? J Am Vet Med Assoc 2004;224(5):676–84.

APPENDIX 1: CLINICAL ETHICS COMMITTEE CONSULT FACILITATION GUIDE

Introduction to process: meeting scheduled at request of _____ to discuss and problem-solve (case) _____, which has triggered several concerns, including concerns about the ethics of continuing care for this patient. Clinical Ethics Committee consults are advisory and intended to help everyone involved in _____ 's care find common ground and construct a workable plan moving forward. We're all here because we care.

REQUIREMENTS

- Consults often involve different opinions about/experiences with the case in question and all viewpoints are valuable. Please be respectful of these differences.
- Solutions are best built on evidence and objective data, so please make sure all statements and concerns are evidence-based.
- In cases where we have concerns about client health and well-being, please avoid diagnostic assertions and instead describe concrete client behaviors and client capacity to consent, to understand illness/treatment, and to adhere.

GUIDING ETHICAL CONSTRUCTS

- Autonomy (on behalf of surrogate decision maker)
- Beneficence (offer and provide care that can plausibly help the patient achieve a reasonable goal; avoid undertreatment or overtreatment and define reasonable outcomes)
- Justice (fairness in distribution of resources, including clinician time)
- Nonmaleficence (first, do no harm)

GUIDING QUESTIONS

- What is the relevant history?
- What are the ethical concerns here? (Can we agree on the core problems?)
- What, if anything, is off the table? (What will we not do, no matter what?)
- What other guidance is necessary (eg, legal, administrative)?
- How might we move forward?

(Form developed by the Clinical Ethics Committee, North Carolina State University-College of Veterinary Medicine)

The Mentor-Mentee Relationship, Addressing Challenges in Veterinary Medicine Together

Yvonne Elce, DVM

KEYWORDS

- Mentor • Mentee • Well-being • Retention • Mosaic

KEY POINTS

- Mentorship in veterinary medicine is currently focused on trainees and early career veterinarians.
- Effective mentor-mentee relationships can contribute to well-being and resilience in veterinarians.
- Mentorship has been shown to play a key role in career progression and retention.
- Veterinary medicine could address many key issues facing the industry by focusing on more substantive and varied mentoring.

INTRODUCTION

The mentor-mentee relationship has existed for many years both informally and formally, although it has been the focus of more research and attention in recent years. Many veterinarians find a mentor early in their education and may keep this mentor for a long period of time.[1] However, mentoring has evolved over time, and because veterinarians face significant challenges it is necessary to examine the relationship and potential for improvement. The relationship has significant beneficial effects both for the mentor and for the mentee. However, as with many things, there is also the potential for abuse and negative effects to occur. In this article, the authors examine the recent research and evidence on mentor-mentee relationships in the context of both the pitfalls of mentorship and the potential benefits. Although a fair amount of literature exists in human medical fields, few studies have examined the effects of mentorship in veterinary medicine. As such, the authors focus on reviewing veterinary literature and refer to the human medical literature when veterinary-specific studies are unavailable.

Veterinary medicine is facing many difficult problems within the profession, but there are efforts to apply mentorship in improving mental health and well-being in

Atlantic Veterinary College, University of PEI, Department of Health management, 550 University Avenue, Charlottetown, PEI Canada C1A 4P3
E-mail address: yelce@upei.ca

Vet Clin Small Anim 51 (2021) 1099–1109
https://doi.org/10.1016/j.cvsm.2021.04.023
vetsmall.theclinics.com

veterinary graduates[2,3]; recruiting public health, emergency medicine, and food animal veterinarians[4]; and in establishing competency.[5] Each of these important issues will be explored as the authors examine the potential to leverage the application of quality mentoring in veterinary medicine. The pitfalls and negatives are explored at the end of the article but it should be noted at the beginning that the quality of evidence for many of the effects of mentoring is fairly low.[6]

DEFINITIONS

To ensure consistency with current literature and throughout the article it is necessary to first define the terms used. The definitions of mentoring vary slightly from article to article but broad common themes are easy to identify. A mentor is defined as a more experienced and knowledgeable person who actively helps guide a less experienced or less knowledgeable person. An advisor is slightly different and often provides advice in a single area or field based on their expertise. A mentor is more encompassing than an advisor and has the goal of allowing the mentee to flourish personally and professionally and develop their own identity. A classic example of this would be a faculty member mentoring a veterinary student, intern, or resident. A mentee is a less experienced or less knowledgeable person who is open to learning and accepting of guidance. Lists of the ideal characteristics of each individual can readily be found in the literature with slight variations.[7] The classic mentor-mentee definition is somewhat strict and does not encompass many other mentoring situations such as mosaic mentoring, group mentoring, or peer-peer mentoring. Peer-to-peer mentoring is one in which the function of the mentor is potentially more supportive although often still slightly more experienced than the mentee. Peer-peer mentoring is often actually cross-age mentoring in which the mentor is of a higher academic level and/or older than the mentee but still within the same social group. An example of this would be a second or third-year veterinary student mentoring a first-year veterinary student. Group mentoring is another concept that could be postulated to address many of the negatives that single mentoring relationships may engender. Group mentoring is defined as having multiple mentors, with each having their unique characteristics and goals. Group mentoring can provide a well-rounded and multifaceted mentoring approach as well as allow various mentor-mentee relationships to exist for short periods when they are required or to acquire new ones as the career of the mentee progresses. This definition overlaps with mosaic mentoring, which is also a term that is being used more frequently with particular emphasis on life-long career progression. Mosaic mentoring has been defined as using multiple and changing or evolving mentors for different life and career needs.

MENTORSHIP AND MENTAL WELL-BEING

Research has demonstrated that effective mentoring can go beyond improving competency,[8] leading to improved well-being for the mentee.[7,9,10] Improved well-being among both veterinary students and graduate veterinarians is of particular concern to a profession with high burnout and suicide rates.[2] One group in the Netherlands examined the effect of a 1-year program for new graduates in veterinary medicine.[2] Although mentoring was not a specific focus, results of the study showed that peer mentoring improved the personal resources of the participants. Improved personal resources are correlated with better coping mechanisms and retention within the profession. It was noted that participants were better able to communicate, which led to improvements in confidence and improved relations with colleagues. These skills were taught in the program, showing that specific interventions can be helpful. A systematic review of near-peer (including overlapping definitions of peer-to-peer or cross-age peer mentoring) mentoring in medical students revealed 3 main outcomes from the mentoring programs for the mentees: improved personal and professional development, stress reduction, and ease of transitioning.[10] In addition, the beneficial effects were not only for the mentee but also for the mentor who experienced positive professional and personal development as well (professional and personal development included improved problem-solving skills, reflective and communication skills, respect, and resilience). This systematic review of the literature encompassed both near-peer mentoring and also multilevel mentoring where faculty mentored senior students who mentored junior students. Use of multilayer mentoring can not only improve personal and professional development in senior students but also ease the time commitment placed on faculty. Peer-to-peer mentoring results seem focused on well-being and resilience with little effect on actual clinical skills.[11] These results again suggest a need to expand on the traditional single-mentor model in the veterinary profession, using mosaic mentoring to allow different individuals to fulfill slightly different, although overlapping, needs of the mentee. The positive effect on mental well-being has been recognized, with many private practices and veterinary corporations taking steps to ensure new graduates have both senior and peer-to-peer mentoring. Both CVS Group PLC and VCA corporate veterinary groups have stated mentoring policies for new graduates, which include establishment of a peer group[a,b].

Mentorship has also been shown to have positive effects on the mentor. It has bidirectional benefits. The pitfalls and potential negatives are discussed later but perceived beneficial effects for the mentor include improved mental well-being with higher self-esteem, personal fulfillment, and enhanced leadership skills.[9] These positive characteristics indicate mentorship may help improve the mental well-being issues present in veterinarians at all levels and bring a greater sense of community.

MENTORSHIP AND COMPETENCY

During the last few years there has been a shift to competency training and assessment in all aspects of veterinary medicine. Competency of a veterinarian includes both professional skills and technical skills. Although there is some evidence that professional skills can be aided through effective mentorship, most of the studies have focused on mentorship and training in the technical skills, as summarized in the following section.

Professional communication in veterinary medicine includes communication with colleagues and members of the team, as well as clients. Studies of well-being in both medical and veterinary students and graduates have noted that increased communication skills can result from targeted mentoring.[2,12] Mentoring is more focused on competency in the domain of professionalism and professional identity, and this has been shown in studies in human medicine with beneficial effects for both mentor and mentee.[9,13] Although improved self-confidence and communication with professional colleagues likely translates into improvement in competency at communication with clients, this effect has not been studied.

Although the effect of mentorship on professional skills has been limited, the effects on technical competency in surgery has been a subject of significant research and can

---

[a] Web site referenced in the text: CVS Group PLC New Graduate Program: https://www.careerswithcvs.co.uk/jobs/roles/graduate-ems-placements.

[b] Web site referenced in the text: VCA new graduate program: https://careers.vcacanada.com/Why-VCA-Canada/Mentorship.

likely be used to extrapolate to other technical competencies. A recent study from New Zealand found that new graduates needed mentoring in surgical skills and required several mentored surgeries before being competent to operate on their own.[5] The number of mentored surgeries required for competency varied depending on type but were basic desexing surgeries (spays and neuters). In human medical training mentorship in surgical training is commonly referenced as being a crucial part of the training.[14–16] The consensus of the Association of Surgeons in Training is that every trainee should have access to a surgical mentor who has been trained in mentorship.[14] The research would suggest this is necessary to ensure competence and patient safety. However, the articles do recognize that the traditional apprentice-ship model is hard to maintain in current working environments due to increased expectations on the mentors. They all recommend training of the mentor and recommend mosaic models with combinations of different mentors for different stages of the career and progression.[7,15,16] Although these studies were performed in human medicine, extrapolation to veterinary medicine would seem valid, due to the similarities of the training programs and skills. Although these articles value mosaic mentoring and can include distance mentoring, there are both safety and technical benefits associated with a same-site mentoring in surgery. Surgical training involves nonvisual cues and physical demonstrations that require in-person contact.[8] Mentor-guided training and intermittent intervention has been shown to significantly improve skills practice and skills competency among mentees.[17] There is certainly sufficient evidence in the literature to support formalized mentoring in veterinary training to improve competency and patient care.

Corporate veterinary groups have taken steps to ensure basic competency with new graduate boot camps and formalized mentorship for new graduates[a,b]. CVS Group PLC has a 3-week summer boot camp for new graduates, including hands-on surgical training and pairing with an on-site practice mentor in addition to peer relationship building. Other veterinary corporate clinics have similar measures. Academic and private practices often have some form of mentoring available; however, it may behoove the veterinary world to have a more formal recommendation as a whole for mentoring in the arena of competency training, not only in surgery but in all competency training. This would demonstrate a global commitment to competency by the veterinary community. Mosaic mentoring is strongly recommended in human medical literature to meet the needs of competency at various levels in an evolving career, and the same is true in veterinary medicine.[7]

There may be some conflict with mentoring and competency in the realm of assessment.[18] Having a mentor seems to be helpful in ensuring competency, particularly in the realm of surgery, but having a mentor involved in the assessment of competency moves from an empowering approach to a more directed approach and may involve some conflicts. Although this effect was not noted in mentor-directed learning,[17] it has been noted in at least one study of mentor-mentee relationships.[18] In veterinary schools with a smaller number of faculty, it is likely that senior mentors may be involved in assessment of the mentee at some point. Having mosaic mentoring with group or peer mentoring may allow this apparent conflict to be avoided, in addition to ensuring that mentors receive training on giving of feedback, reflection, and empowering the learner.

MENTORSHIP AND RETENTION AND RECRUITMENT

Recruitment and retention of veterinarians in certain areas of the profession are acknowledged problems in veterinary medicine.[3,19–21] Mentoring has been recognized as a valid method of improving retention and recruitment in business and medical disciplines, but few studies have been performed in veterinary medicine.[1,22,23] There has been more recent veterinary literature on the mentorship of veterinarians in their first job positions after graduation, which has been performed in New Zealand and North America.[3,19,20] Although the importance of finding a position with a positive mentor during the early stages of the career is emphasized as crucial to retention within the profession, there are few studies that provide evidence regarding practices that improve retention. An article looking at mentoring in one midwestern state showed that having a mentor improved career success and that the mentor was frequently from their first job experience.[1] Two studies performed in Canada showed that a lack of mentorship increased the chances of a veterinarian moving away from their first job and away from food animal practice.[19,20] A more recent study looked at the experiences of recent veterinary graduates in New Zealand and why they may have left their first job.[3] A toxic work culture and a lack of mentorship were the 2 main reasons graduates left their employment.[3] New graduates stated that having an employer who checked in regularly and gave regular feedback was an important characteristic to their mental well-being (both are known characteristics of an effective mentor). In England a large survey in 2020 has been performed with BEVA (British Equine Veterinary Association) and BSAVA (British Small Animal veterinary Association), which also shows that the team culture is crucial for retention as well as regular feedback[c]. Both the article from New Zealand and the recent survey in the United Kingdom show that almost half of the veterinarians are considering a job change in the next 1 to 2 years.[3,c] These retention issues can to a large degree be addressed through mentoring. Several institutions and associations have started programs to address these very concerns. BEVA has a "Leg Up" program where new graduates are paired with more experienced practitioners who have undergone advanced training in coaching and mentoring[d], and this provides a distance mentor that is beneficial to new graduates and would be best if a mentor from the same practice also existed to create a mosaic mentoring situation. Mosaic mentoring is presumed to have benefits in that one mentor may be more suited to aid in decisions about career progression, another for actual competency mentoring being physically present for some procedures, and another for personal or interpersonal issues. BEVA provides voluntary participation in this program and also provides Mumsvet[e], which provides support for young professionals with families (regardless of gender despite the name). The combination of these programs starts to promote new graduates to have a mosaic of mentors and in the future studies should be performed to analyze the effect of this program. CVS Group PLC, which is a corporation that owns many practices in the United Kingdom and Europe, has a new graduate program that not only provides the summer camps for competency training but also pairs new graduates together for peer support as well as a trained "clinical buddy" at the practice site for on-site mentoring[a]. Again, this scheme uses both peer mentoring and classic mentoring to try and create a support network that enables new graduates to survive and thrive in clinical practice. VCA in North America offers mentorship for the first 90 days in practice to help with the transition for new graduates, and many other corporations offer similar promises of mentorship and support[b]. The fact that the largest

---

[c] Web site referenced in the text: BEVA and BSAVA recruitment and retention survey. Renate Weller and colleagues https://www.beva.org.uk/retention-survey.

[d] Web site referenced in the text: BEVA Leg Up program: https://www.beva.org.uk/CPD-and-Careers/Career-Coaching.

[e] Web site referenced in the text: BEVA Mumsvet program: https://www.beva.org.uk/CPD-and-Careers/MumsVet.

forces in corporate veterinary medicine are investing resources and time in mentorship programs serves as an additional evidence of the recognized value of these efforts in retention and recruitment of new veterinarians. However, controlled studies that document the effects and potential drawbacks of these programs are lacking at this time.

Specific veterinary groups have also looked at mentoring as a method of recruitment into areas of veterinary medicine where it has proved to be particularly difficult to attract and retain veterinarians. Emergency veterinary medicine has been studied, and fear of a lack of mentoring was identified as a specific deterrent to entering into this area.[24] The same effect has been identified in food animal practice.[19,20] Ironically, the paucity of veterinarians in each of these areas often leads to recruitment of new graduates into single veterinarian practices where in-person mentorship would be impossible. Mentoring has also been shown to increase the number of veterinary students going into internships[21] and is important for recruiting vets into academia, comparative medicine, public health, and food animal medicine.[4] Although studies in the use of mentorship programs for recruitment into certain fields are rare in veterinary medicine, evidence in the human medical literature suggests that mentorship has been effective, particularly with the use of mosaic mentoring.[23]

MENTORSHIP AND DIVERSITY

Although there are no studies of the interaction between mentorship and diversity in the veterinary literature, information from studies performed in other health-related fields suggests that mentorship may be important in addressing issues of diversity in veterinary medicine.

Gender

In the human medical field, studies on the influence of gender in mentoring have demonstrated varying results.[13,23,25] Although gender may be important for some in the mentor-mentee relationship it was not important for all individuals or for all situations. As a result, mosaic mentoring has been used to allow gender-specific mentoring in certain areas, while allowing non–gender-specific mentoring in other areas such as skill acquisition.[23,25] Use of mosaic mentoring, group mentoring, and peer mentoring was helpful in reducing the mentoring workload on few available faculties in one specific gender. A study of women in rural health care settings with limited mentors used a diverse group of mentors from both academia and corporate worlds, finding that the combination was valuable and allowed diverse perspectives to the mentee.[26] Although the veterinary profession is much more feminized than human medical professions, some areas remain less changed[27,28] and so consideration of gender may still be important in the veterinary milieu for both men and woman. It is stated that being able to "see" people similar to yourself (in gender, for example) is likely more important than having your mentor be similar to yourself, but this has not been fully studied appropriately.[23]

Diversity

Although a limited number of studies have examined the importance of gender in mentoring, the effect of differences in culture or race is even less known. As veterinary schools seek to improve diversity this may become an important topic for concern. Lack of mentors from underrepresented backgrounds or overload of the few faculty available may have negative impacts. The stated mechanisms for dealing with a low number of female mentors may be applied to the lack of availability of diverse mentors to avoid overwhelming those few faculty members. Lack of mentors who are similar to the mentees in terms of culture and ethnicity has been seen as a systematic failure in the human medical field and a barrier to improving diversity,[13] although the scientific evidence is limited. Training can also be used to improve mentoring across differences and diminish unconscious bias.[29,30] A study examining mentor's experiences with communication to mentees of different cultures revealed that cultural differences can be a stumbling block in the relationship. Empathy was noted to be crucial in overcoming differences, and training on intercultural competence was recommended.[30] Training in cross-culture differences and overcoming unconscious bias would improve communication between mentor and mentee and help overcome a lack of diverse mentors currently available in veterinary medicine. Unfortunately, both medical education and mentorship within surgical education have been identified as possessing ethical issues with prejudice against women and ethnic minorities, so programs that involve mentorship should be monitored to ensure prejudice and poor attitudes are not tolerated.[6,31,32]

Generational Differences

Finally, generational differences can serve as a barrier to effective communication between mentors and mentees.[16] Mosaic mentoring may help obviate problems across different generations, with peer mentoring and senior mentors bringing different attributes to the conversation. Online mentoring has been increasingly studied and may be used more readily by younger generations. Distance mentoring has been traditionally effective in research fields,[33] and online mentoring is the natural technological evolution of this, allowing time and distance to become less of a barrier. This may also aid in increasing diversity by allowing access to diverse mentors and mentees globally. The drawbacks noted were that the distance created a sense that the mentor was an outsider and potentially less competent to help, whereas increased availability and flexibility as well as less hierarchical feeling were benefits.[34]

NEGATIVES ABOUT MENTORING

Mentoring is, at its base, about excellent communication, and when it goes poorly, there is the potential for temporary breakdowns and even failures. Mentoring is frequently associated with a more senior person in a position of some influence that is interacting with a person of lower rank or seniority, creating a power dynamic the potential for abuse.

Unfortunately, although mentoring relationships have clear potential to cause harm, there are few validated, robust instruments available to evaluate mentorships and diagnose problems.[35] Furthermore, the few mentor assessment tools that have been developed are not in widespread use.[36] Given the potential damage that can result from inadequate or outwardly negative mentoring relationships, practices should regularly evaluate the efficacy of mentoring within their team and make changes where needed.

No article specifically studies the rates of abuse in mentor-mentee relationships in veterinary contexts. Information in other medical fields suggests that common pitfalls include limited access to mentors, unrealistic expectations, lack of time on the part of the mentors, lack of career reward for the mentors, and lack of training.[37,38] A systematic review of mentorship in medical surgical training found similar common ethical issues among different studies, namely negative attitudes, failure of communication, lack of respect and disturbingly, prejudice again women, and ethnic minorities.[6] This article also identified issues on the part of the mentee and the institution as well as giving potential solutions. Well-managed and designed mentoring programs can avoid these generic pitfalls. Limited numbers of available mentors can be leveraged at each institution by using a variety of mentoring types (peer-to-peer, mosaic, distance mentoring). Unrealistic expectations should be avoided through clear communications and may result from limited numbers and time on the part of the mentors. Clear guidelines on what to expect should be established at the beginning of each mentoring relationship. Expectations may vary from place to place and should be explicit. Setting expectations enables not only availability to be set but guidelines on what the relationship is for and what the roles will be. Mentors may try to mold mentees into themselves and control rather than facilitate mentees to develop their own identities. Use of mentees to achieve the mentors' own goals for professional advancement is difficult to monitor, as promoting the career progression often involves mentored projects and achievement of goals. Having monitoring of the mentor program is highly recommended as well a clearly defined method of ending the relationship.[35]

Verbal, physical, and sexual harassment can and do occur. Although most institutions have reporting mechanisms for these problems, some do not and it should be explicit in the beginning of mentoring relationships that there are mechanisms for ending the relationship particularly with traditional mentor-mentee relationships. Having group or mosaic mentoring helps prevent these pitfalls, as the mentee has other people to talk to and to recognize potential abusive behaviors. Peer-to-peer mentoring can help a mentee identify when a behavior is not in line with what other mentees have experienced and is protective. Periodic confidential surveys may help monitor the levels of harassment within a system while acknowledging and highlighting its importance. Training of mentors would also help mentors develop the skills necessary to become effective mentors and avoid some pitfalls.

Abusive relationships have been described in studies of the medical school training environment.[39] Questionnaires distributed to graduating medical students by the American Association of Medical Colleges have specific questions regarding abusive situations, although not specific to mentoring.[39] Indeed the findings of some of these articles would suggest that the problems identified concerning diminishing well-being could be significantly helped by mentoring at all stages of a career, as they stem less from actual abuse and more from interactions with unhappy senior residents or faculty. This syndrome of unhappy senior clinicians also exists in veterinary medicine and likely contributes to attrition and lack of employee retention as well as abuse in mentoring relationships.[40] Significant rates of sexual violence are also reported in human medical school studies.[41] Importantly these studies have led to active methods to improve the environment and reduce mistreatment.[31] Although the veterinary environment may differ significantly from the human medical learning environment, issues in diversity and equality still exist,[28] and further study on when and how much mistreatment occurs is a crucial step that needs to be taken. There are number of articles addressing stress in veterinary students but without reference to abuse of power specific to mentoring, and so monitoring programs need to be established. Confidential surveys of students such as those described in medical schools would allow the information on abuse to be collected and the conversation about discrimination to be informed.

SUMMARY

Mentorship currently occurs in many forms in the veterinary field although research into the topic is limited. Based on the literature available in both veterinary and medical fields, mentorship has the potential to address some of the existential crises facing veterinary medicine today. Using mentorship in various forms may be one tool in the toolkit available to tackle these important issues and promote joy in the veterinary profession. Some private practice employers and organizations are starting to advertise mentorship programs as a method for recruitment and retention, and most veterinary schools have formalized mentorship programs for students, house officers, and faculty. There is a distinct need for broader studies on the current use of mentors and their benefits and negatives as well as prospective studies on new forms of mentoring and use of mosaic and peer-to-peer mentoring in the veterinary world. Integration of peers and seniors in an evolving fashion would seem to be able to facilitate the growth and development of veterinarians on both sides of the mentoring equation. There is also a clear need for negative issues to be acknowledged and addressed with information gathering and analysis to aid in preventative measures being developed against abuse in the future. It would behoove the profession to address these issues as a whole rather than individual institutions and practices. Veterinary medicine globally needs thoughtful and deliberate mentoring at all stages to enable veterinarians and their clients and patients to benefit from competent, empathetic, and joyful veterinarians.

DISCLOSURE

No funding was provided for this article, and there are no conflicts of interest to declare.

REFERENCES

1. Niehoff BP, Chenoweth P, Rutti R. Mentoring within the veterinary medical profession: veterinarians' experiences as proteges in mentoring relationships. J Vet Med Educ 2005;32(2):264–71.
2. Mastenbroek NJJM, van Beukelen P, Demerouti E, et al. Effects of a 1 year development programme for recently graduated veterinary professionals on personal and job resources: a combined quantitative and qualitative approach. BMC Vet Res 2015;122:311.
3. Gates MC, McLachlan I, Butler S, et al. Experiences of recent veterinary graduates in their first employment position and their preferences for new graduate support programmes. N Z Vet J 2020;68(4):214–24.
4. Freeman LC. Rx for recruitment and retention of veterinarian scientists: money, marketing, mentoring. J Vet Med Educ 2005;32(3):328–36.
5. Gates MC, Littlewood KE, Kongara K, et al. Experience of practicing veterinarians with supervising final year students and new graduates in performing desexing surgeries. J Vet Med Educ 2020;47(4):465–73.
6. Lee FQH, Chua WJ, Cheong CWS, et al. A Systematic scoping review of ethical issues in mentoring in surgery. J Med Educ Curricu Dev 2019;6:1–13.
7. Singletary SE. Mentoring surgeons for the 21st century. Annals Surg Oncol 2005;12(11):848–60.
8. Sutkin G, Littleton EB, Kanter SL. How surgical mentors teach: a classification of in vivo teaching behaviours part 2: physical teaching guidance. J Surg Educ 2015;72(2):251–7.
9. Toklu HZ, Fuller JC. Mentor-mentee relationship: a win-win contract I graduate medical education. Cureus 2017;5(9):e1908.
10. Akinla O, Hagan P, Atioma W. A systematic review of the literature describing the outcomes of near-peer mentoring programs for first year medical students. BMC Med Educ 2018;18:98.

11. Altonji SJ, Banos JH, Harada CN. Perceived benefits of a Peer Mentoring Program for First Year Medical Students. Teach Learn Med 2019;31(4):445–52.
12. Van Patten RR, Bartone AS. The impact of mentorship, preceptors and debriefing on the quality of program experiences. Nurse Educ Pract 2019;35:63–8.
13. Henry-Noel N, Bishop M, Gwede CK, et al. Mentorship in medicine and other health professions. J Canc Educ 2019;34:629–37.
14. Sinclair P, Fitzgerald FD, McDermott FD, et al. Mentoring during surgical training: Consensus recommendations for mentoring programmes from the Association of Surgeons in Training. Editorial Int J Surg 2014;12:S5–8.
15. Patel VM, Warren O, Ahmed K, et al. How can we build mentorship in surgeons of the future? ANZ J Surg 2011;81:418–24.
16. Entezami P, Franzblau LE, Chung KC. Mentorship in surgical training: a systematic review. Hand 2012;7:30–6.
17. Aho JM, Ruparel RK, Graham E, et al. Mentor-guided self-directed learning affects resident practice. J Surg Educ 2015;72(4):674–9.
18. Meeuwissen SNE, Stalmeijer RE, Govaerts M. Multiple-role mentoring: mentors' conceptualisations, enactments and role conflicts. Med Educ 2019;53:605–15.
19. Jelinski MD, Campbell JR, MacGregor MW, et al. Factor associated with veterinarians' career path choices in the early postgraduate period. Can Vet J 2009; 50:943–8.
20. Jelinksi MD, Campbell JR, Naylor JM, et al. Factor associated with the career path choices of veterinarians in western Canada. Can Vet J 2009;50:63–636.
21. Barbur L, Shuman C, Sanderson MW, et al. Factors that influence the decision to pursue an internship: the importance of mentoring. J Vet Med Educ 2011;38(3): 278–87.
22. Cochran A, Paukert JL, Scales EM, et al. How medical students define surgical mentors. Am J Surg 2004;187(6):698–701.
23. Bettis J, Thrush CR, Slotcavage RL, et al. What makes them different? An exploration of mentoring for female faculty, residents, and medical students pursuing a career in surgery. Am J Surg 2019;218:767–71.
24. Booth M, Rishniw M, Kogan LR. The shortage of veterinarians in emergency practice: A survey and analysis. J Vet Emerg Crit Care 2020;1–11. https://doi.org/10.1111/vec.13039.
25. Welch JL, Jimenez HL, Walthau J, et al. The women in emergency medicine mentoring program: an innovative approach to mentoring. J Grad Med Educ 2012; sept:362–6.
26. Wozniak TM, Miller E, Wiliams KJ, et al. Championing women working in health across regional and rural Australia- a new dual-mentorship model. BMC Med Educ 2020;20:299.
27. Colopy SA, Buhr KA, Bruckner K, et al. The intersection of personal and professional lives for male and female diplomates of the American College of Veterinary Surgeons in 2015. J Am Vet Med Assoc 2019;255(11):1283–90.
28. Morello SL, Colopy SA, Bruckner K, et al. Demographics, measures of professional achievement, and gender differences for diplomates of the American College of Veterinary Surgeons in 2015. J Am Vet Med Assoc 2019;255(11):1270–82.
29. Osman NY, Gottlieb B. Mentoring across differences. MedEdPORTAL 2018;14: 10743.
30. Hagqvist P, Oikarainen A, Tuomikoski AM, et al. Clinical mentors experiences of their intercultural communication competence in mentoring culturally and linguistically diverse nursing students: A qualitative study. Nurse Educ Today 2020;87: 104348.

31. Pradhan A, Buery-Joyner SD, Page-Ramsey S, et al. To the point: undergraduate medical education learner mistreatment issues on the learning environment in the United States. Am J Obstet Gynecol 2019;Nov:377–82.
32. Fnais N, Soobiah C, Chen MH, et al. Harassment and discrimination in medical training : a systematic review and meta-analysis. Acad Med 2014;89(5):817–27.
33. Falcone JL, Croteau AJ, Schenarts KD. The role of gender and distance mentoring in the surgical education research fellowship. J Surg Educ 2014;72(2):330–7.
34. Dorner H, Misic G, Rymarenko M. Online mentoring for academic practice: strategies, implications and innovations. Ann N Y Acad Sci 2021;1483:98–111.
35. Ng YX, Koh ZYK, Yap HW, et al. Assessing mentoring: A scoping review of mentoring assessment tools in internal medicine between 1990 and 2019. PLoS One 2020;15(5):e0232511.
36. Yukawa M, Gansky SA, O'Sullivan P, et al. A new mentor evaluation tool: evidence of validity. PLoS One 2020;15(6):e0234345.
37. Burgess A, van Diggele C, Mellis C. Mentorship in the health professions: a review. Clin Teach 2018;15:197–202.
38. Collins H. Mentoring veterinary students. J Vet Med Educ 2005;32(3):285–9.
39. Slavin SJ, Chibnall JT. Mistreatment of medical students in the third year may not be the problem. Med Teach 2017;39(8):891–3.
40. Moore IC, Coe JB, Adams CL, et al. The role of the veterinary team effectiveness in job satisfaction and burnout in companion animal veterinary clinics. J Am Vet Med Assoc 2014;245(5):513–24.
41. Moreno-Tetlacuilo LMA, Quezada-Yamamoto H, Guevara-Ruisenor ES, et al. Gender-based relations and mistreatment in medical schools: A Pending agenda in mexico and the world. Gac Med Mex 2016;152:726–31.

Communicating Patient Quality and Safety in Your Hospital

Beth Davidow, DVM

KEYWORDS

- Quality • Patient safety • Psychological safety • Just culture • Medical errors
- Adverse events • Model for improvement

KEY POINTS

- Quality must be defined before it can be discussed. Safety, timeliness, efficiency, effectiveness, equity, and patient/pet family centeredness are important components of quality medicine.
- Human hospitals with the best patient outcomes have cultures that emphasize continuous improvement and interdepartmental communication.
- Patient safety is improved in hospitals in which team members feel safe in openly discussing mistakes, making suggestions, and speaking up when concerned.
- Using a formalized 6-step process can improve outcomes for patients, clients, and staff when a medical error occurs.

WHAT IS QUALITY?

Many of us intuitively know what quality is. However, it can be hard to communicate what quality care involves unless we take the time to think deeply and define it. There are many definitions of quality. Merriam-Webster has definitions of quality that include, "a degree of excellence," and "superiority in kind."[1] The Oxford Learners Dictionary defines quality as "the standard of something when it is compared to other things like it."[2] The American Society for Quality defines quality in business more specifically as "characteristics of a product or service that bear on its ability to satisfy stated or implied needs" and "a product or service free of deficiencies."[3]

Human medicine started understanding the impact that deficiencies had on quality care in the late 1990s. A 1998 study found that medication errors (**Box 1**) were responsible for at least 7000 deaths.[4] This report led the Institutes of Medicine to form the Committee on the Quality of Healthcare in America. Their 2000 report, *To Err is Human*, confirmed the huge toll of mistakes and estimated that actually between

Veterinary Clinical Sciences, Washington State University, 205 Ott Road, Pullman, Washington, DC 99163
E-mail address: Elizabeth.davidow@wsu.edu

Vet Clin Small Anim 51 (2021) 1111–1123
https://doi.org/10.1016/j.cvsm.2021.04.019
vetsmall.theclinics.com
0195-5616/21/© 2021 Elsevier Inc. All rights reserved.

> **Box 1**
> **Definitions**
>
> Medical error: A commission or an omission with potentially negative consequences for the patient that would have been judged wrong by skilled and knowledgeable peers at the time it occurred, independent of whether there were negative consequences.[23]
>
> Medication error: A medical error involving a medication.
>
> Adverse event: Untoward medical occurrence in a patient undergoing a treatment or receiving a medication, which may be either preventable or not preventable.[36]
>
> Near miss: Medical error that results in no harm to the patient.[5]
>
> Psychological safety: Being able to show and employ one's self without fear of negative consequences of self-image, status, or career.[37]
>
> Forward accountability: The ability to learn from an account to prevent future mistakes.[33]

44,000 and 98,000 Americans died each year as a result of medication errors.[5] This report was a wake-up call that despite the best efforts of the health care system, in many instances there was more harm than health.

The publication of *To Err is Human* led to the passage of the Healthcare Research and Quality Act. This legislation tasked the American Health Quality Association (AHQA) with providing annual reports on quality. Owing to the impact of errors on quality, it stipulated that adverse events must be reported by any hospital that received Medicare/Medicaid reimbursement.

The publication of *To Err is Human* was followed in 2001 by *Crossing the Quality Chasm*.[6] In this report, the Institutes for Medicine identified other defects, in addition to medical errors (see **Box 1**), that were threats to quality health care. The committee proposed 6 aims for improvement that they believed would address the key dimensions of quality. To be high quality, health care should be:

Safe: avoiding errors that harm patients.
Timely: reducing waits and delays for needed care.
Effective: providing services based on current scientific understanding and avoiding both under- and overuse.
Efficient: avoiding waste of equipment, supplies, energy, and so on.
Equitable: providing care that does not vary in quality because of geography, gender, ethnicity, or socioeconomic status.
Patient centered: ensuring that patient values and preferences guide the care received.

In 2008, to further put the onus on hospitals to improve care, the Centers for Medicare and Medicaid services began denying hospitals higher payment for hospital care that was complicated by hospital-acquired conditions including catheter-related urinary tract infections and patient injury due to falls.[7] The ethical and financial considerations have led to concerted efforts to prevent errors, and this has led to overall system improvements. From 2010 to 2014, there was 17% reduction in hospital acquired conditions. Data from 2014 to 2017 showed a further 13% decrease.[8] Despite these decreases in hospital-acquired conditions, a 2016 study estimated that deaths in the United States due to all medical errors were likely 250,000 per year, putting it as the third leading cause of death in the country.[9]

We can use information from *To Err is Human* and *Crossing the Quality Chasm* to craft and discuss what quality means in veterinary medicine. As in human medicine, a discussion of quality in veterinary medicine must start with an understanding of whether our service is "free of deficiencies" or errors. Safety must come first. Timeliness, efficacy, efficiency, and equity are as important in veterinary as in human medicine. Patient centered is crucial for human medicine, whereas quality in the veterinary realm may be best when it is pet family centered, with the families' values, preferences, and abilities at the forefront when care decisions are made for the pet.

To pull these concepts together, I communicate quality veterinary medicine as safe, reliable, and effective health care that puts pets and their families first.

SAFETY FIRST: UNDERSTANDING ERRORS IN VETERINARY MEDICINE

How common are medical errors in the veterinary field? There is no overall reporting or screening process for errors in veterinary medicine. However, studies are starting to reveal that errors are a threat to quality in our profession. A 2018 survey study of veterinarians regarding medical errors received 606 responses. Of those responding, 73.8% reported involvement in at least one near miss or adverse event.[10] A study of adverse event reporting at Cornell University over 3 years showed a medical error incidence rate of 5 of every 1000 visits; 85% were no-harm events, whereas 15% did result in harm and 8% resulted in permanent harm or death.[11] Although small, these studies indicate that we need more research in understanding the prevalence and causes of errors in veterinary practice.

CULTURE MATTERS

Quality can vary dramatically between health care locations. The 2020 Watson Health top 15 health system study demonstrated that there is 15% lower incidence of complications, 12.5% lower incidence of hospital-acquired conditions, and 3.8% fewer deaths in the top human health care systems compared with other health groups studied. In addition, top hospitals had 10% shorter hospital stays.[12]

A 2011 study examined why differences in quality exist. The researchers studied the reasons behind differences in mortality from acute myocardial infarction in human hospitals in the top and bottom 5% in outcome ratings.[13] The researchers interviewed more than 150 staff at 11 hospitals, 7 with the highest survival and 4 from the lowest. There were clear common themes differentiating the top and bottom performers. Employees in the top hospitals reported that there was a common, visible commitment from leaders to providing high-quality, exceptional care. The employees also reported that adverse events were used as opportunities to learn and that input was gathered from all levels of the organization for solutions. It was reported that nurses and doctors were held accountable to high standards and were engaged in overall quality improvement efforts. In addition, there was an emphasis on smooth communication flow between departments. Last, these hospitals had a commitment to using clinical guidelines, standard order sets, and specific discharge planning. Thus it was found that culture, rather than equipment, technology, or facilities, had the biggest impact on outcome.

A 2016 study had similar findings. The study was originally looking for differences in outcome based on geographic location and examined 22 million inpatient hospitalizations across the country. The investigators found that there was a 10-fold difference in patient safety outcomes, an 18-fold difference in catheter infection rates, and a 2-fold difference in overall mortality between the top and bottom decile hospitals. Geography was not predictive of outcome, and they also found that individual hospital culture was most likely responsible for the quality differences.[14]

Google spent 2 years interviewing its employees to understand the differences between the highest and lowest performing teams in their organization. It was hypothesized that having the right balance of technical skills would be critical to success. However, after looking at many attributes and interviewing more than 200 employees, they discovered that cultural factors were most predictive of success. These factors were similar to those found in the hospitals with the best outcomes: meaning and impact of work was understood; there was psychological safety, structure, and clarity; and the team could depend on one another.[15]

CREATING CULTURE

Creating a culture of excellence thus starts with a clear mission that safety and quality matter (**Box 2**). In the myocardial infarction study, employees at top hospitals described their mission as "the glue," and "the driving force behind everything."[13] Another employee described this pursuit of excellence: "[We are] constantly resetting that bar. . . . [I]f you aim for As, you get As, and if you accept Zs, that's what you get. We don't accept anything less than the very best."[13]

Similarly, The Mayo Clinic states that, "in order to be trusted, we must be safe"; they communicate this culture by a written commitment to safety that is part of their orientation for students, house officers, and new physicians.[16]

Thus it is critical that your mission and core values reflect a commitment to quality and safety. This commitment should be incorporated into onboarding for new staff and new veterinarians. Staff meetings, ongoing hospital training, and written memos are also ways to communicate your mission and why safe practices lead to improved outcomes for pets.

Psychological safety (see **Box 1**) can be defined simply as the belief that you will not be punished when you speak up or make a mistake. Teams are much more likely to learn about mistakes and problems in workflow when they feel safe speaking up. When blame is replaced by curiosity, you can develop *"forward accountability,"* the ability to learn from an account to prevent future mistakes.

To create psychological safety, leaders must commit to asking people to speak up if they are concerned and then must thank them when they do[17]; this is especially important for client care representatives, janitorial staff, assistant, and technical staff. These staff members are on the frontline of care and often identify risks early. Risks could include a cage door that does not latch easily or an autoclave that sometimes does

---

Box 2
Incorporating quality and safety into hospital culture

1. Include a commitment to safety in your onboarding and training materials.

2. Provide clear and easy ways for staff members to provide suggestions; this might include suggestion boxes, apps, online forms, and/or open discussion at regular meetings.

3. Start a routine of a 5-to-10-minute daily huddle to organize the day and alert everyone to any possible patient concerns.

4. Create an improvement board (or internal webpage) that lists projects in process or tracks improvement

5. Develop a patient safety reporting system and use it to guide improvement projects

6. Celebrate quality improvement project successes (and the people who help)

7. Discuss cases that did not proceed as planned in the spirit of forward accountability

not heat up all the way. When people feel safe bringing up concerns, safety issues come to the forefront before they lead to harm.

Phrases can be taught to staff to communicate a possible safety risk. In the case of a medication dosage that might be too high, they could say, "I need a little clarity – can you explain this dose to me. It seems higher than what I have seen used before." If they are worried that a pet may undergo respiratory arrest with a procedure, they could try, "I am concerned about taking radiographs on this patient given how hard they are breathing." If they do not feel their concerns are heard, they could escalate the language to, "I feel taking radiographs right now on this patient is unsafe."

There are other ways to signal that you want input. Visible suggestion boxes, online suggestion forms, or electronic communication channels devoted to employee ideas are all ways to gather ideas for improvement. Directly asking for volunteers to help brainstorm a solution to a safety concern also builds engagement, especially if you are willing to try a creative proposed solution. It is critical to respond to suggestions with gratitude. Acting on suggestions is also crucial to show that you are listening and willing to implement change for improvement.

Instituting a routine daily huddle is another way to establish a culture of communication and commitment to safety. A daily huddle is a 5- to 10-minute stand-up meeting that can occur at the start of a work shift. The purpose of the meeting is to check in at the start of the day and allow a space to bring up any safety or specific patient concerns for the day. It can also be a chance to provide thanks for hard work or a specific action the day before.

Importantly, creating culture is about not only what you say but also what you do. If you say you want your staff to speak up but then get angry when they tell you about a situation that did not go smoothly, they will stop speaking up.

STRUCTURE AND CLARITY

Providing health care is complex, and this complexity is one reason why errors occur. Human medicine has realized that one way to make sure that clinical practice matches published evidence-based guidelines is to implement order sets and checklists. The Surviving Sepsis Campaign has made pocket cards to emphasize the initial steps in care that need to happen within 1 hour if sepsis is suspected.[18] Studies in both human and veterinary medicine have shown that implementing a surgical checklist can decrease postoperative complications.[19–22] Checklists can be used in other parts of veterinary hospitals to avoid missing key elements of important processes. The use of hospital-specific guidelines and checklists can provide clarity on expectations for care.

RESPONDING TO A MEDICAL ERROR

The way we deal with medical errors is one of the strongest ways to communicate our core beliefs about quality and safety (**Box 3**). In addition, studies in human health care and veterinary medicine have shown that the way we respond to serious medical mistakes affects the outcome of the patient, the likelihood of legal action by the client, and the long-term resilience of the health care team.[13] The way we respond may also affect the opinion of other veterinarians and the community.

Health care team members involved in an error are likely to feel a combination of emotions including fear, guilt, defensiveness, and denial. It is important to acknowledge these emotions while responding to an adverse event and finding long-term solutions. The following 6-step process provides a framework for response in the case of an adverse event or medical error.

> **Box 3**
> **Six-step response to medical errors**
>
> 1. Treat the patient first
> 2. Notify the client promptly
> 3. Support the veterinary staff involved
> 4. Investigate
> 5. Circle back to the client
> 6. Fix internal systems

The Patient Should Always Come First

As soon as a mistake, error, adverse event, or potential side effect is noted, care should be taken immediately to minimize ongoing damage, to fix or support body systems, and to get help as needed to improve the chances of a good outcome. In the case of an inadvertent drug delivery or overdose, contacting a poison hotline such as the American Society for the Prevention of Cruelty to Animals® (ASPCA) is recommended. In the case of a surgical mistake, consulting with a surgical specialist early should be strongly considered. A local specialty hospital or teaching hospital could also be consulted. The Veterinary Information Network and other online resources may also be sources of information about overdoses or unpublished treatment side effects.

Notify the Client Right away

Health care providers should be aware of the ethics associated with disclosure of errors. Do you tell clients of every mistake or near miss even if there is no harm? What if the error happened but the patient already had a grave prognosis? What if the error was made by another veterinarian?

There is strong agreement in human health care that any error resulting in serious harm must be disclosed to the patient.[23] In research focus groups, most patients say they want to be informed of all mistakes, even if no harm resulted.[24–26]

Many legal cases occur when people feel that the medical team is not being honest because they do not feel that improvement is going to occur. Studies in the human field have shown that disclosure reduces the intent to sue, reduces the size of awards if a case goes to court, and discourages plaintiff attorneys from taking these cases.[27–29] In 36 states, a statement of apology or sympathy is not admissible in a human malpractice case if it is made quickly after an event.

Clients specifically want explicit acknowledgment that an error occurred; they want to know exactly what the error was and if there are any clinical implications. Clients want to know WHY the error happened and how recurrences will be prevented. Most importantly, they want a sincere apology and empathy from the team.[26]

The language and timing are both important. Initially, describe only what facts you know, not what you assume. In some cases, you may not know why the pet is doing poorly. Immediately let the client know that their pet's health is your first concern and that you are treating them while investigating. Let them know WHEN you will give them more information, WHO will call them, and then STICK to your promise on communication timing. It is important to sincerely express sympathy, support, and concern. Do not blame specific people because this is often seen as shirking responsibility and undermines the team. The phrase "I'm so sorry this happened," expresses empathy and may be most appropriate until a full investigation can be performed to truly understand what happened.

Disclosure is one of the hardest parts of what we do. In a 2004 study of US and Canadian doctors about disclosure, 74% said it was very difficult. Many doctors chose their words carefully and often did not explicitly identify the error or discuss how to prevent recurrence.[30]

Being mentally prepared for these conversations is important. Many clients will be angry, may yell, and may request to speak to a different doctor or your supervisor. Discussing scenarios like these ahead of time helps the situation go more smoothly.

If the mistake happens when a practice owner or supervisor is not available, it is always best to say, "We are going to do everything we need to care for XX. The medical director/practice manager/owner have been notified and will be in contact with you as soon as possible after reviewing the case." Veterinarians are most likely to handle disclosure well if they understand the protocol and expectations. A script and written information for disclosure is extremely useful. Role playing for physicians has been shown to improve communication in these situations.[31]

A program at the University of Michigan was implemented that worked to make sure all harmful errors were disclosed quickly and appropriately and to compensate patients quickly and fairly. Over 5 years, the number of lawsuits dropped by 50%, the time to resolve claims dropped in half, and litigation costs dropped by two-thirds.[28,29] This program is now published as a training module available online.[32]

Support the Health Care Workers Involved

No one wants to make a mistake. Most of us are in veterinary medicine because we love animals and want to help, not hurt. In addition, many in health care are perfectionists who work extremely hard to be accurate and many already have self-doubt. It is important to deal with the situation at hand without blame. Asking, "Are you OK?" is crucial for healing.

A study of 32 shelter veterinarians who had an adverse event occur in spay-neuter surgeries showed that the response of the team to the event was crucial for allowing the veterinarian to process, to learn from the event, and to continue to practice. The veterinarians who received support and collegiality, perspective and appraisal, and technical learning and emotional learning were more likely to move on and become resilient.[27]

It is often asked whether there is ever a time when a staff member should be held responsible or even fired. The concept of "just culture" can be key in looking at this question. The essence of "just culture" is that health care workers who make an honest mistake, even (or especially) one that results in severe patient harm, require support rather than punishment. We should presume that everyone is trying to do their best for the patient and to improve quality. Our job is to provide an environment where it is easy to do the right thing and harder to do the wrong thing.

Investigate

Investigation is needed to provide a full accounting to the owner and to understand options for prevention. The first glance "why" is usually not the full story. Asking why multiple times can lead you toward a root cause. Investigation should be centered on forward accountability (see **Box 1**) and "just culture."[33] Four questions can be asked. First, did the staff member cause the harm deliberately? As stated earlier, this is almost never true, but if it were, consequences would be appropriate. If not deliberate, then was the staff member drunk, high, or otherwise impaired at work? If the answer to this question is yes, then substance abuse help is needed. If neither of these are true, then does the staff member have a history of mistakes that cannot be explained? In this case, the specific roles or tasks may not be appropriate. The last and potentially most important question is whether another person in the same situation could have made the same mistake; this is often true and why it is so important to look closely at why the mistake occurred. When investigating, ask what was responsible for the incident versus who was responsible.[33]

For example, a common serious adverse event in veterinary hospitals is patient burns from heat sources that are applied during or after an anesthetic procedure. It may seem like it was the "fault" of a veterinary team member who heated a hot water bottle too much or used an electric heating pad inappropriately. However, owing to the frequency of reported burns, we know that the heat sources themselves are inherently unsafe. Thus the safest response is removal of electric heating pads and hot water bottles from veterinary hospitals, not blame or reprisal toward a staff member.

Another example is demonstrated in a study from University of Florida (Buckley GJ, Eide M, Sanchex LC, et al. The effect of implementation of standardized medication order writing on dosing errors in a referral hospital. J Vet Emerg Crit Care 2018; 28(S1): S27-S35). A technician gave a dose of medication at 10 mg rather than 10 mg/kg that was ordered. It would be easy to say that the technician should read orders more carefully. However, because University of Florida was tracking and categorizing medication errors, they demonstrated that many medication errors were happening due to misinterpretation of orders. On further investigation, they found that clinicians ordered medications in different ways, sometimes in mg/lb, sometimes in milliliters, sometimes by tablet. As there was no standard, it could be easy to misinterpret a milligram dose as a mg/lb or mg/kg dose. By agreeing as a hospital to a set medication ordering protocol, medication errors due to misinterpretation were significantly decreased. Fixing the system rather than just talking to individual staff members improved safety (Buckley GJ, Eide M, Sanchex LC, et al. The effect of implementation of standardized medication order writing on dosing errors in a referral hospital. J Vet Emerg Crit Care 2018; 28(S1): S27-S35).

Circle Back to the Client

Although it is important to inform the client about a potential medical error right away, it is impossible to give them a full answer until the pet is stable, experts are consulted, and an investigation is performed. Clients need closure and a full story so setting a time to discuss your findings and your ongoing plan is important. A time for a second discussion should be set not long after the initial event but with enough time to prepare appropriately.

Work to Fix Systems Internally

The only thing worse than dealing with a medical error is dealing with the same medical error repeatedly. Creating a process to report, track, and investigate all medical errors (with and without harm) will allow you to know what mistakes happen and to start the process of continuous improvement.

Crossing the Quality Chasm states, "Trying harder will not work. Changing systems of care will. Poor designs set the workforce up to fail, regardless of how hard they try."[6] To look for system changes, human health care quality improvement has embraced, The Model for Improvement.[34] This system provides a roadmap for asking questions, brainstorming possible solutions, and then testing a proposed change. The idea is to test improvements scientifically but at a faster pace than a standard research study.

The goal is to find solutions that ideally create no additional work for staff members. We want to minimize complexity and cost whenever possible. Thus, it is important to discard changes that do not work so that we only use what actually helps to make patient care safer. Three questions can help to start an improvement process.

QUESTION 1: WHAT ARE WE TRYING TO ACCOMPLISH?

By clearly stating what we are trying to do, it is easier to develop a concrete goal, plan, and metric to see if you have been successful. Examples of possible goals might be (1) reduce time from admission to seeing the emergency room doctor to an average of 60 minutes, (2) decrease the number of cats with a urinary tract infection post urinary catheter by 50%, or (3) report all laboratory work within 1 business day.

QUESTION 2: HOW WILL WE KNOW THAT A CHANGE IS AN IMPROVEMENT?

If you can find something to measure, it is easier to tell if you have fixed or improved the problem; this may involve making sure you know what your baseline is to start. It is also important to find a way to measure that is doable on the timeframe that makes sense. For wait times, you may be able to use your computer software or an intensive care unit flow sheet program. For secondary urinary tract infections or reporting laboratory work, you may need a data tracking system.

QUESTION 3: WHAT CHANGE CAN WE MAKE THAT WILL RESULT IN IMPROVEMENT?

It is important to involve your team in brainstorming possible changes. If your suggested change is unworkable or disliked, it will not be fully implemented. Ideas can be generated through brainstorming sessions, through reading, through surveys of other hospitals, or by looking at other industries. In general, the staff most involved in the process may have the most ideas for improvement.

PDSA CYCLES

A Plan-Do-Study-Act (PDSA) cycle is a way to think of getting the ball rolling.

- *Plan:* This is simply naming what change you are going to try. In general, change happens best when we start with a small change in a small setting. If you are in a large hospital and you wonder if creating a medication order form will help minimize errors, it may work best to start it as a trial on one day of the week or just in one department.
- *Do:* Try the change for a set time.
- *Study*: Decide what you are going to measure and when you are going to measure
- *Act*: If the change was not successful, stop, brainstorm, and try again with a new plan. If it was successful on a small scale, this is the time to try it on a larger scale; this may mean rolling out the change to another department, another day of the week, or another time of day.

EFFECTIVENESS OF SAFETY CHANGES

Not all improvements are equal. Improvements that focus on individuals, improving training, or reminding people to be more careful, are weak forms of improvement. Checklists and written policies that make it easy to do things correctly and harder to do them incorrectly provide stronger improvement. The most effective, although often most challenging to implement, are changes that make it impossible to do the task incorrectly. Examples include syringes that only fit certain drugs to avoid incorrect administration and needleless systems to eliminate the risk of needle sticks. These changes are highly effective but can require infrastructure changes and have associated costs. Many common improvement projects fall somewhere in the moderately effective category.

Once an improvement plan is identified, it needs to be rolled out. Buy-in from people affected by the policy is critical, and without buy-in, the policy will not be successful. The PDSA cycle provides an effective model for implementation of improvement projects and provides data that you can then use to demonstrate effectiveness to your team. You will need to have a good system for both rolling out new policies and then making sure these policies are easily accessible. Employees are frustrated if they are in violation of a policy they did not know existed.

MEDICATION SAFETY

Medication errors are the most common type of mistake in health care. Anticipating that these errors can happen and using training to help prevent these errors can be a good first area to improve in a veterinary hospital.

The 6 rights of medication administration should be emphasized to all new employees (including veterinarians). These 6 rights to check every time a medication is given include right patient, right drug, right dose, right route, right time, and right documentation. Including these in your training checklists and posting this list in pharmacy can help emphasize that medication safety is part of your culture.

Another way to decrease the likelihood of medication error is to minimize the use of verbal medication orders. Training assistants and technicians to only give medications that are written down avoids errors due to mishearing (15 vs 50, Convenia vs Cerenia). There are situations, such as cardiopulmonary resuscitation, surgery, or treatment of an actively seizuring patient, where written orders are not feasible. In those situations, using closed loop communication is key. Closed loop communication involves the receiver repeating back the order and waiting for confirmation. For example, "Give 0.5 mL epinephrine IV," "I'm giving 0.5 mL epinephrine IV," "Correct."

Double check systems are another way to prevent medication errors. The system may be that all new employees must have medications checked before administering for the first month of employment and/or that insulin, sedatives, and chemotherapeutic drugs must always be double checked before administering. Writing initials on prescription labels, both the person who made the prescription and then the doctor before sending home, is yet another double check that decreases the risk of an error.

MOTIVATING PROGRESS AND CELEBRATING WINS

Visual documentation of improvement can be a great way to motivate your hospital. Improvement in health care feels daunting owing to the size and scope of our caseloads. Being able to break down issues and problems into manageable chunks and then showing that some headway is being made can encourage folks to keep working on the first issue and even find, define, and tackle a new area.

Improvement boards (**Fig. 1**) are used in many health care organizations to let everyone know the projects that are being worked on and progress that is being made. The boards differ in type, size, and what is shown. Some hospitals have room for suggestions, whereas others are very data driven with many charts and graphs. Having some type of display or area specifically reserved for discussion of improvement helps to prioritize its importance in your hospital.

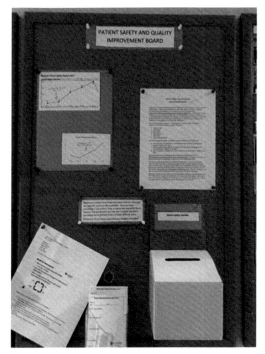

Fig. 1. Example of an improvement board and suggestion box.

SUMMARY

Communication and culture are key to improving quality and patient safety in your practice. An emphasis on mission, psychological safety, and continuous improvement is critical for improving patient outcomes. A report on hospital quality and improvement strategies suggested that one of the most important steps is to "be patient but unrelenting, recognizing that change takes time and quality must continually be kept on the front burner."[35]

DISCLOSURE

The author has no conflicts of interest.

REFERENCES

1. Merriam-Webster. Quality. 2021. Available at: https://www.merriam-webster.com/dictionary/quality. Accessed March 30, 2021.
2. Oxford University Press. Quality. 2021. Available at: https://www.oxfordlearnersdictionaries.com/us/definition/english/quality_1. Accessed March 30, 2021.
3. American Society of Quality. Quality Glossary. 2021. Available at: https://asq.org/quality-resources/quality-glossary/q. Accessed March 30, 2021.
4. Phillips DP, Christenfeld N, Glynn LM. Increase in US medication-error deaths between 1983 and 1993. Lancet 1998;351(9103):643–4.
5. Kohn L, Corrigan J, Donaldson M. To Err is human. Washington, DC: National Academies Press; 2000.

6. Institute of Medicine (US) Committee on Quality of Health Care in America. Crossing the quality Chasm: a new health system for the 21st Century. Washington, DC: National Academies Press (US); 2001. Available at: https://www.ncbi.nlm.nih.gov/books/NBK222271/. Accessed March 30, 2021.

7. Levinson DR. Adverse events in hospitals: national incidence among Medicare beneficiaries. Department of Health and Human Services; 2010. Available at: https://oig.hhs.gov/oei/reports/OEI-06-09-00090.pdf. Accessed March 31, 2021.

8. Agency for Healthcare Research and Quality. AHRQ National Scorecard on Hospital-Acquired Conditions Final Results for 2014-2017. Rockville, MD. 2020. Available at: https://www.ahrq.gov/sites/default/files/wysiwyg/professionals/quality-patient-safety/pfp/Updated-hacreportFInal2017data.pdf. Accessed March 31, 2021.

9. Makary MA, Daniel M. Medical error-the third leading cause of death in the US. Br Med J 2016;353:i2139.

10. Kogan LR, Rishniw M, Hellyer PW, et al. Veterinarians' experiences with near misses and adverse events. J Am Vet Med Assoc 2018;252(5):586–95.

11. Wallis J, Fletcher D, Bentley A, et al. Medical Errors Cause Harm in Veterinary Hospitals. Front Vet Sci 2019;6:1–7.

12. IBM Watson Health. Watson Health 15 Top Health Systems Study. Cambridge, MA. 2020. Available at: https://www.ibm.com/downloads/cas/GDBBYRWE. Accessed March 31, 2021.

13. Curry LA, Spatz E, Cherlin E, et al. What distinguishes top-performing hospitals in acute myocardial infarction mortality rates? Ann Intern Med 2011;154(6):384–90.

14. Rosenberg BL, Kellar JA, Labno A, et al. Quantifying Geographic Variation in Health Care Outcomes in the United States before and after Risk-Adjustment. PLoS One 2016;11(12):e0166762.

15. Rozovsky J. re:Work - the five keys to a successful Google team 2015. Available at: https://rework.withgoogle.com/blog/five-keys-to-a-successful-google-team/. Accessed March 31, 2021.

16. Mayo Clinic Health System. Provider Orientation. 2013. Available at: https://www.mayoclinichealthsystem.org/~/media/Local Files/Waycross/Documents/ProviderOrientationOnline.pdf. Accessed March 31, 2021.

17. Delizonna L. High -performing teams need psychological safety. Here's how to create it. Harvard Business Review. 2017. Available at: https://hbr.org/2017/08/high-performing-teams-need-psychological-safety-heres-how-to-create-it. Accessed March 31, 2021.

18. Surviving Sepsis Campaign. Surviving Sepsis Campaign - Adult Patients. 2021. Available at: https://www.sccm.org/SurvivingSepsisCampaign/Guidelines/Adult-Patients. Accessed March 31, 2021.

19. Cray MT, Selmic LE, McConnell BM, et al. Effect of implementation of a surgical safety checklist on perioperative and postoperative complications at an academic institution in North America. Vet Surg 2018;47(8):1052–65.

20. Menoud G, Axiak Flammer S, Spadavecchia C, et al. Development and Implementation of a Perianesthetic Safety Checklist in a Veterinary University Small Animal Teaching Hospital. Front Vet Sci 2018;5:3.

21. Haynes AB, Weiser TG, Berry WR, et al. A surgical safety checklist to reduce morbidity and mortality in a global population. N Engl J Med 2009;360:491–9.

22. Bergström A, Dimopoulou M, Eldh M. Reduction of surgical complications in dogs and cats by the use of a surgical safety checklist. Vet Surg 2016;45(5):571–6.

23. Wu AW, Cavanaugh TA, McPhee SJ, et al. To tell the truth: Ethical and practical issues in disclosing medical mistakes to patients. J Gen Intern Med 1997; 12(12):770–5.

24. Fein SP, Hilborne LH, Spiritus EM, et al. The many faces of error disclosure: A common set of elements and a definition. J Gen Intern Med 2007;22(6):755–61.

25. Dudzinski DM, Hébert PC, Foglia MB, et al. The disclosure dilemma — large-scale adverse events. N Engl J Med 2010;363(10):978–86.

26. Gallagher TH, Waterman AD, Ebers AG, et al. Patients' and physicians' attitudes regarding the disclosure of medical errors. J Am Med Assoc 2003;289(8):1001–7.

27. White SC. Veterinarians' emotional reactions and coping strategies for adverse events in spay-neuter surgical practice. Anthrozoos 2018;31(1):117–31.

28. Kachalia A, Kaufman SR, Boothman R, et al. Liability claims and costs before and after implementation of a medical error disclosure program. Ann Intern Med 2010;153(4):213–21.

29. Adams MA, Elmunzer BJ, Scheiman JM. Effect of a health system's medical error disclosure program on gastroenterology-related claims rates and costs. Am J Gastroenterol 2014;109(4):460–4.

30. Gallagher TH, Waterman AD, Garbutt JM, et al. US and Canadian physicians' attitudes and experiences regarding disclosure errors to patients. Arch Intern Med 2006;166:1605–11.

31. Etchegaray JM, Gallagher TH, Bell SK, et al. Error Disclosure Training and Organizational Culture. 2017. Available at: https://www.ncbi.nlm.nih.gov/books/NBK508075/. Accessed March 31, 2021.

32. Aqency for Healthcare Research and Quality. Communication and optimal resolution (CANDOR). Available at: https://www.ahrq.gov/patient-safety/capacity/candor/index.html. Accessed March 31, 2021.

33. Dekker S. Just culture: restoring trust and accountability in your organization. 3rd edition. Boca Raton: CRC Press, Taylor and Francis Group; 2017.

34. Langley G, Moen R, Nolan K, et al. The improvement guide. 2nd edition. San Francisco, CA: Josey-Bass; 2009.

35. Alteras T, Meyer J, Silow-Carroll S. Hospital performance improvement: trends in quality and efficiency—a quantitative analysis of performance improvement in U.S. Hospitals | Commonwealth fund 2007. Available at: https://www.commonwealthfund.org/publications/fund-reports/2007/apr/hospital-performance-improvement-trends-quality-and-efficiency?redirect_source=/publications/fund-reports/2007/apr/hospital-performance-improvement-trends-in-quality-and-efficiency-a-qua. Accessed March 31, 2021.

36. CFR - Code of Federal Regulations Title 21. Available at: https://www.accessdata.fda.gov/scripts/cdrh/cfdocs/cfcfr/cfrsearch.cfm?fr=312.32. Accessed March 31, 2021.

37. Kahn WA. Psychological conditions of personal engagement and disengagement at work. Acad Manag J 1990;33(4):692–724.

Printed and bound by CPI Group (UK) Ltd, Croydon, CR0 4YY

03/10/2024

01040477-0007